Anti-Epileptic Drug
Interactions:
A Clinical Guide

Anti-Epileptic Drug Interactions: A Clinical Guide

P. N. PATSALOS

Institute of Neurology
National Hospital for Neurology and Neurosurgery
Queen Square, London
and
The National Society for Epilepsy
Chalfont St Peter
United Kingdom

Published by

Clarius Press Ltd
8 Holly Lea, Guildford,
Surrey GU4 7PG, United Kingdom

Copyright © 2005 by Clarius Press Ltd

British Library Cataloguing in Publication Data
A catalogue record for this book is available from the British Library

ISBN 09542279-5-6

Produced by Wellset Repro Ltd, Cranleigh, United Kingdom

FOREWORD

Drug interactions can be a major complication in the clinical management of epilepsy. There are many reasons for this: (i) although monotherapy is solidly established as the therapeutic mainstay, combinations of antiepileptic drugs (AEDs) continue to be widely prescribed in patients who did not respond to a single drug; (ii) because of the chronic nature of epilepsy treatment, the likelihood of AEDs being co-administered with other drugs for the management of associated or intercurrent conditions is considerable; (iii) many AEDs are potent inducers or inhibitors of drug metabolising enzymes, and they are highly likely to modify the pharmacokinetics of concurrently administered agents; (iv) most AEDs have a narrow therapeutic index, and even modest changes in their plasma drug concentration can result in seizure breakthrough or signs of toxicity.

Over the years, our understanding of AED interactions has increased greatly, but the sheer size of available data has discouraged many clinicians from taking an effective approach to minimize the adverse consequences which may result from these interactions.

Philip Patsalos, a leading expert in this area, has to be commended for his successful effort to put together a massive amount of information in a concise and easily accessible format. Anti-Epileptic Drug Interactions: A Clinical Guide is divided into four sections:

- a general introduction which explains the basic mechanisms of drug interactions and tools to make predictions about their occurrence;
- a directory which allows immediate identification of what interactions are to be expected when any of the available AEDs is combined with other AEDs;
- a directory of AED interactions affected by specific agents grouped within therapeutic classes, e.g. antimicrobials, cardiovascular drugs, psychotropic drugs, herbal remedies, and so on;
- a directory of interactions whereby specific agents, grouped within therapeutic classes, are affected by AEDs.

This publication provides an invaluable tool for consultation by the practising clinician. Not only does it give immediate information on the probability that interaction-related changes in response occur when another drug is added or discontinued, but it also explains what magnitude of change can be anticipated and what steps may be taken to minimize adverse consequences. An added useful feature is that, in addition to specifying which drugs cause interactions, other drugs within the same therapeutic class for which no interactions occur are also listed. This helps the physician in making rational drug choices by identifying therapeutic alternatives which are less likely to cause problematic interactions.

Two caveats need to be highlighted when using this guide. The first is that, as the author correctly acknowledges, interactions are often subject to prominent interindividual variability: the magnitude of change in blood levels which is listed in this publication generally reflects the maximum effect that can be anticipated, but it should in no way be taken as the most accurate prediction of the degree of interaction which will occur in the individual patient. The second caveat is that the compilation focuses on pharmacokinetic drug interactions, and we have to be aware that at times clinically important changes in response result from pharmacodynamic interactions, i.e. interactions where no changes in total or unbound plasma levels can be identified. To keep the publication within an easily handled format, the author elected not to provide specific references for the many interactions described. In an era where the Internet allows immediate retrieval of literature sources, this should not detract from the general usefulness of this work.

By keeping this publication on their desk (or in their pocket), physicians can now count on an additional tool for rational prescribing, eventually resulting in improved quality of care of their patients.

Emilio Perucca, MD, PhD, FRCP(Edin)

Professor of Clinical Pharmacology, University of Pavia, Italy
Director, Laboratories for Diagnostics and Applied Biological Research,
Institute of Neurology IRCCS C. Mondino Foundation, Pavia, Italy.

Disclaimer

PREFACE

The purpose of this book is to provide in a systematic fashion a description of the most clinically relevant drug interactions that occur between AEDs and between AEDs and non-AEDs, which may present problems for patients with epilepsy and that frequently require therapeutic adjustment. With this information it is anticipated that physicians will be better placed so as to allow a more rational drug choice when polytherapy regimens are indicated and, also, to allow for a more informed rationale as to how drugs will interact and, therefore, the dosage adjustment that would be consequently necessary so as to maintain an appropriate therapeutic response.

The book is divided into four colour-coded sections:

- **the Introduction** explains the basic mechanisms of drug interactions, how to anticipate and predict interactions and how to prevent and manage adverse interactions;

- **Section 1** describes the interactions that occur between AEDs;

- **Section 2** describes interactions that occur between AEDs and non-AED drugs whereby the interaction affects AEDs. The non-AED drugs are listed in drug classes;

- **Section 3** describes interactions that occur between AEDs and non-AED drugs whereby the interaction affects non-AED drugs. The non-AED drugs are listed in drug classes.

While the focus of this book is on pharmacokinetic interactions, pharmacodynamic interactions are equally important and are therefore highlighted where appropriate. As a drug class, the number of known AED interactions is substantial, and whilst it has been the author's aim to be as complete as possible, the listings may not be exhaustive and the possibility exists that clinically significant interaction will occur with other drugs.

The data used in compiling this guide were identified by searches of Medline and PubMed with the terms "antiepileptic drug interactions" combined with individual drug names and drug groups, references from relevant articles, and searches of the author's files. No gender or age limits were imposed but searches, last conducted April 2005, were limited to human subjects (healthy volunteers or patients and included case reports) and to in vitro data. Only papers published in English were reviewed and abstracts were reviewed only when a complete published article was not available. Because physicians treating patients with epilepsy are very familiar with drug blood levels and how changes in these levels are reflective of a drug's pharmacokinetic characteristics and efficacy/adverse effect profile, the pharmacokinetic interactions presented in this book are described in terms of a change in blood levels. However, in some studies blood levels are not reported and instead clearance, half-life, area under the concentration versus time curve (AUC) and/or maximum blood level (Cmax) values are quoted. Thus, for these studies, the interactions are described in terms of changes in clearance, half-life, AUC and/or Cmax values. Whenever available, pharmacokinetic changes in mean values are quoted; otherwise a value representing the most significant change reported, for example in small case series, is quoted. Finally, some studies do not quote any pharmacokinetic variables and instead describe the interaction in terms of a change in the clinical status (enhanced/reduced therapeutic response or enhanced toxicity) of the patient. For these interactions, the interactions are described generically, for example "enhances the metabolism" or "inhibits the metabolism" of the affected drug. Wherever the data are available, interactions are also described in relation to their effects on hepatic enzyme activity, for example, cytochrome P450, uridine glucuronyl transferases and epoxide hydrolase, so as to allow the reader to ascertain the propensity of similar interactions occurring with other drugs that may have similar enzyme activities as substrates, inhibitors and/or inducers.

When using the information detailed in this book, the reader should remember that although a drug interaction is considered clinically relevant when it results in the need for dosage adjustment or other medical intervention in the majority of patients, a marked deviation in an unusually susceptible individual is also important. Also, one needs to consider the end result because a marked elevation in a low AED/drug level may improve seizure control/therapeutic response whilst a small elevation of a nearly toxic level may actually precipitate toxicity. Finally, whilst an interaction involving a 10% change in a drug blood level may have little, if any, clinical relevance in the majority of patients it may be of profound clinical relevance in some patients.

Philip N Patsalos

London, June 2005

CONTENTS

Introduction

Epilepsy is a chronic disorder, which is primarily treated with antiepileptic drugs (AEDs) that are usually prescribed for prolonged periods and often for a lifetime. The older long- established generally available AEDs (carbamazepine, ethosuximide, phenobarbital, phenytoin, primidone and valproic acid) can render approximately 80% of newly diagnosed patients seizure-free when administered as monotherapy regimens. For the remaining 20% of patients, the prescribing of polytherapy (2 or more drugs) AED regimens so as to achieve optimal seizure control is a common practice. However, for the majority of these patients little additional benefit is achieved from the use of polytherapy AEDs as intolerable adverse effects commonly occur as a consequence of pharmacokinetic and/or pharmacodynamic interactions. Furthermore, for those patients that respond to monotherapy, they too may experience the consequences of AED interactions as AEDs are added and withdrawn during the optimisation of their monotherapy drug regimen. A further confounding factor is that since epilepsy is a chronic condition many patients will inevitably develop comorbid diseases or other debilitating conditions and disorders, which will require the co-administration of non-AED drugs. In this setting the potential for drug interactions is considerable. A further source of potential clinically significant interactions that is being increasingly recognised relates to the increasing use of over-the-counter medications and supplements, many of which have unknown constituents. Finally, AEDs are increasingly used to treat other non-epilepsy conditions such as mood disorders, migraine and pain, thereby further increasing the possibility of combined use with other drugs.

The pharmacokinetic properties of AEDs make them particularly susceptible to drug interactions. Furthermore, many of the older long-established AEDs have a narrow therapeutic index in that the plasma (serum) level (concentration) associated with a desirable antiepileptic effect is close to the plasma level that is associated with undesirable adverse effects. Thus, even a relatively small change in their plasma level (due to inhibition or induction) may readily result in signs of intoxication or loss of seizure control. In addition, some AEDs exert a major influence on the activity of hepatic drug metabolising enzymes, stimulating (e.g. carbamazepine, phenytoin, phenobarbital and primidone) or inhibiting (e.g. valproic acid) their activity thereby leading to a wide variety of interactions with other drugs that are also metabolised and eliminated by the same enzymes. Conversely, because most AEDs undergo extensive hepatic metabolism, they too are vulnerable to the effect of other drugs with inhibiting or inducing properties. In the clinical setting, an important objective of AED treatment is to anticipate and minimize the risks of interactions with other agents. An unexpected loss of seizure control or development of toxicity during AED therapy often accompanies the addition or removal of a concurrently administered drug. This propensity for clinically relevant drug interactions with AEDs relates to their chronic administration, narrow therapeutic index, involvement of hepatic metabolism in their elimination, and the ability of several AEDs to enhance or inhibit the hepatic metabolism of other drugs.

Mechanisms of drug interaction

There are two basic types of drug interaction:

1. Pharmacodynamic interactions

These interactions, which occur between drugs that have similar or opposing pharmacological mechanisms of action, take place at the cellular level where drugs act. Consequently, although pharmacodynamic interactions are important, they are less well recognised since they are not associated with any change in plasma drug level. Thus, these interactions are usually concluded by default whereby a change in the clinical status of a patient consequent to a drug combination cannot be ascribed to a pharmacokinetic interaction.

2. Pharmacokinetic interactions

These involve a change in the absorption, distribution, metabolism or elimination of the affected drug and consequently alter levels (concentrations) at the site of drug action. These interactions comprise most of the interactions reported and are associated with a change in plasma level of either the drug or its metabolite(s) or both.

Pharmacodynamic interactions

Although pharmacodynamic interactions have been traditionally neglected in epilepsy therapy, increasing evidence indicates that their recognition is essential so as to maximise AED efficacy and minimise AED toxicity. Most pharmacodynamic interactions simply involve additive neurotoxicity, and may be explained by superimposition of adverse events caused by AEDs sharing the same modes of action. For example, combinations of two sodium-channel blockers, such as carbamazepine and oxcarbazepine, or carbamazepine and lamotrigine, are less well tolerated than combinations of drugs acting through different mechanisms. Combinations of drugs that enhance GABAergic inhibition, such as valproic acid and phenobarbital, may result in profound sedation that cannot be explained solely by a pharmacokinetic interaction. Lamotrigine and valproic acid in combination may produce disabling tremor. Examples of potential favourable drug combinations include: valproic acid and ethosuximide (in the management of refractory absence seizures) and valproic acid and lamotrigine (in the management of partial and generalised seizures).

Pharmacodynamic interactions between AEDs and non-AED drugs can also result in increased toxicity. For example, there is some evidence to suggest that the increased incidence of neurotoxicity associated with lithium and carbamazepine in combination is primarily the consequence of a pharmacodynamic interaction. Also, the concurrent use of lithium and valproic acid has been associated with additive adverse reactions such as weight gain, sedation, gastrointestinal complaints and tremor. Finally, combining carbamazepine with clozapine is generally contraindicated due to concerns about potential additive adverse haematological side effects.

Pharmacokinetic interactions
Interactions affecting drug absorption

Interactions affecting the absorption of AEDs are uncommon, although occasionally they can be important. For example, antacids reduce the absorption of phenytoin, carbamazepine and gabapentin. Furthermore, phenytoin absorption is impaired when the drug is given together with certain nasogastric feeds (e.g. Isocal) so that plasma phenytoin levels are reduced by 72%. In both examples it is thought that the formation of insoluble complexes may be responsible for the reduced absorption.

Plasma protein binding displacement interactions

Interactions involving protein-binding displacement are important only with the highly protein-bound (>90%) AEDs (e.g. phenytoin, tiagabine and valproic acid). Because these drugs have a low intrinsic hepatic clearance, their displacement causes an initial transient increase in total drug plasma level prior to re-equilibration and a subsequent decrease. However, there is no change in the non-protein bound (free), pharmacologically relevant level, and thus the clinical effects of the AED should also be unchanged. Thus, no adjustment in dose is usually necessary following displacement of highly protein-bound AEDs (e.g. the displacement of phenytoin by valproic acid) from plasma protein binding sites. It is important, however, to recognize that the clinical effects of the AED will now correspond to lower total plasma levels and patient management may benefit from monitoring free non-protein bound drug levels.

Interactions at the renal level

Interactions at the level of renal elimination can be expected to occur with drugs that are predominantly renally eliminated and indeed such clinically relevant interactions have been described (e.g. quinidine, amiodarone and verapamil appear to decrease the renal clearance of digoxin). In relation to AEDs, gabapentin, levetiracetam, pregabalin and vigabatrin are primarily eliminated by renal excretion; however, to date an effect on their renal elimination by concomitant drugs has not been reported.

Metabolic interactions

By far the most clinically significant pharmacokinetic interactions with AEDs are those related to changes in hepatic metabolism and involve induction or inhibition of drug metabolism (Table 1). With the exception of gabapentin, levetiracetam, pregabalin and vigabatrin, all AEDs undergo hepatic metabolism and consequently are susceptible to inhibitory and/or induction interactions. Metabolic processes serve to convert a drug into one or more metabolites, which are more water-soluble than the parent drug and thus facilitate urinary excretion. These processes are catalysed by various enzyme systems, which can occur in series, and are referred to as Phase I (functionalization) and Phase II (conjugation) enzyme systems. Phase I reactions include hydroxylation (the addition of a polar functional group) or N-demethylation (deletion of a non-polar alkyl group) by oxidation, reduction or hydrolysis. Phase II reactions serve to further increase the water solubility of the drug/metabolite and involve conjugation with glucuronic acid, sulphate, acetate, glutathione or glycine. Although metabolic drug interactions may involve changes in any one of the numerous enzymes involved in drug metabolism, by far the most important are those associated with the cytochrome P450 system (CYP). The importance of the CYP system stems from the fact that it is not only responsible for the oxidative metabolism of many drugs and exogenous compounds but also of many endogenous compounds such as prostaglandins, fatty acids and steroids.

CYP enzymes

The CYP enzyme system consists of a superfamily of isoenzymes that are located in the smooth endoplastic reticulum, primarily in the liver but also in many other tissues (e.g. intestine, kidney, brain and placenta). They are classified into families

Introduction

(the first Arabic number; there is a >40% amino acid sequence identity within family members), subfamilies (the capital letter that follows; there is a >59% amino acid sequence identity within subfamily members) and individual isoenzymes (the second Arabic number). Although in man approximately 60 different CYP isoenzymes have been identified, five isoenzymes (CYP3A4, CYP2D6, CYP2C9, CYP1A2 and CYP2C19) are known to be responsible for the metabolism of 95% of all drugs, and three (CYP2C9, CYP2C19 and CYP3A4) are of particular importance in relation to AED interactions. Because the activity of these

Table 1: Antiepileptic drug effects on hepatic enzymes

Drug	Effect	Enzymes affected
Carbamazepine	Induction	CYP2C, CYP3A, CYP1A2, EH and UGT
Clobazam	None	-
Clonazepam	None	-
Ethosuximide	None	-
Felbamate	Induction Inhibition	CYP3A4 CYP2C19, ß-oxidation
Gabapentin	None	-
Lamotrigine	None/weak inducer	UGT
Levetiracetam	None	-
Oxcarbazepine	Induction (weak)	CYP3A4, UGT
Phenobarbital	Induction	CYP2C, CYP3A, EH, UGT
Phenytoin	Induction	CYP2C, CYP3A, EH, UGT
Pregabalin	None	-
Primidone	Induction	CYP2C, CYP3A, EH, UGT
Tiagabine	None	-
Topiramate	Induction (weak) Inhibition (weak)	CYP3A4, - oxidation CYP2C19
Valproic acid	Inhibition	CYP2C9, EH, UGT
Vigabatrin	None	-
Zonisamide	None	-

CYP=cytochrome P450; EH=epoxide hydrolase (microsomal); UGT=uridine glucuronyl transferases

isoenzymes is genetically determined, genetic polymorphism resulting in enzyme variants with higher, lower or no activity, or even resulting in the absence of an isoenzyme can have a profound effect on the pharmacological expression of an interaction (vide infra). In relation to AEDs, those polymorphisms that have clinical consequences relate primarily to CYP2C9 and CYP2C19.

Epoxide hydrolases

Epoxide hydrolases are a family of enzymes whose function is to convert arene oxides to trans-dihydrodiols and simple epoxides to vicinal diols by hydration and consequently are involved in detoxification processes, although sometimes they are involved in bioactivation reactions. Only the microsomal form of epoxide hydrolase is involved in xenobiotic metabolism and plays an important role in the metabolism of carbamazepine, phenobarbital and phenytoin. Epoxide intermediates have been implicated in teratogenic events and hypersensitivity reactions and in relation to the epoxide metabolite of carbamazepine (carbamazepine-10,11-epoxide) it has been implicated in various important interactions (e.g. valproic acid inhibits activity and phenobarbital enhances activity).

Uridine glucuronyl transferases

In humans, three families of uridine glucuronyl transferases (UGTs) have been identified, of which UGT1 and UGT2 appear to be the most important in drug metabolism. The UGT1A3 and UGT2B7 isoforms are involved in the O-glucuronidation of valproic acid and UGT1A4 has been found to be the major isoform responsible for the metabolism (N-glucuronidation) of lamotrigine. Although any substrate of UGT has the potential to competitively inhibit the glucuronidation of other substrates by the same isoform, there are few data in this regard. Furthermore, unlike the CYP system, no specific UGT inhibitors have been identified. Nevertheless, valproic acid inhibits several UGTs whilst carbamazepine, phenobarbital and phenytoin are inducers (e.g. interactions with lamotrigine).

Enzyme induction

Primarily enzyme induction is the consequence of an increase in enzyme protein resulting from an increase in gene transcription that is mediated by intracellular receptors. However, enzyme induction may also occur by an inducer-mediated decrease in the rate of enzyme degradation, through stabilisation of proteins, as occurs with ethanol induction. Thus, although there are several different mechanisms of enzyme induction, the phenobarbital "type" has been best characterised. Indeed, even though phenobarbital is the prototype enzyme-inducing drug, many other drugs (e.g. carbamazepine, phenytoin, primidone and rifampicin) also enhance drug metabolising enzymes with induction patterns that overlap that of phenobarbital. The enzymes associated with phenobarbital "type" induction include CYP1A2, CYP2B6, CYP2C8, CYP3C9 and CYP3A4, epoxide hydrolase and some UGTs.

The resultant elevated enzyme activity, consequent to enzyme induction, results in an increase in the rate of metabolism of the affected drug, leading to a decrease in plasma level and possibly a reduction in the therapeutic response. If the affected drug has a pharmacologically active metabolite, induction can result in increased metabolite levels and possibly an increase in drug toxicity. The amount of enzyme induction is generally proportional to the dose of the inducing drug. As enzyme induction requires synthesis of new enzymes, the time course of induction (and indeed the reversal of induction upon removal of the inducer) is dependent on the rate of enzyme synthesis and/or degradation and the time to reach plasma steady-state levels of the inducing drug. The latter is usually the rate-limiting step and only occurs at a time which is ~ 5 elimination half-lives of the inducing drug. Thus, the time course of induction is usually gradual and dose-dependent.

Enzyme induction represents a common problem in the management of epilepsy. Phenobarbital, carbamazepine and phenytoin are potent inducers of CYPs, although phenytoin and carbamazepine appear to be less potent inducers at doses used clinically. The elderly appear to be less sensitive than younger adults to inducers and thus there is reduced induction of drug metabolism in the elderly, although the evidence for this is contradictory. The reason for the age-dependent response to inducers is not fully understood. Although enzyme induction generally reduces the pharmacological effect of a drug because of increased drug metabolism, sometimes the formed metabolite has the same pharmacological activity as the parent drug. Thus, the clinical consequence of enzyme induction will be determined by the relative reactivity of the parent drug and the formed pharmacologically active metabolite.

Of the AEDs presently used in clinical practice carbamazepine, felbamate, oxcarbazepine phenobarbital, phenytoin, primidone and topiramate at doses of ≥ 200 mg/day are the only drugs that are associated with clinically important hepatic enzyme inducing properties.

Introduction

Enzyme inhibition

Enzyme inhibition is the consequence of a competition by drugs to bind to the same enzymic site resulting in a reduction of enzyme activity and a decrease in the rate of metabolism of the affected drug. Inevitably plasma levels are elevated and this is commonly associated with clinical toxicity. Inhibition is usually competitive in nature and therefore dose-dependent and tends to begin as soon as sufficient levels of the drug inhibitor are achieved, and this usually occurs within 24 hours of inhibitor addition. The time to maximal inhibition will depend on the elimination half-life of the affected drug and the inhibiting agent. When the inhibitor is withdrawn, the time course of de-inhibition is dependent on the elimination half-life of the inhibitor. Among the AEDs valproic acid, topiramate and felbamate have been associated with inhibitory interactions. Furthermore, whilst topiramate and felbamate are primarily selective inhibitors of CYP2C19, valproic acid is considered to be a broad-spectrum inhibitor of hepatic metabolizing enzymes as it inhibits CYP2C9, UGTs and microsomal epoxide hydrolase.

In some circumstances inhibitory interactions are complicated and problematic. For example, interactions involving the active metabolite(s) of the co-administered drugs may not always be obvious if concurrent plasma level changes of the parent drug do not occur. Because it is not common practice to monitor plasma metabolite levels, if one is unaware of the interaction, blood level monitoring of the parent drug could be misleading. Such problematic interactions are associated with carbamazepine-10,11-epoxide, the pharmacologically active metabolite of carbamazepine. For example, during valproate and carbamazepine combination therapy, patients can experience adverse effects as a result of an elevation of carbamazepine-10,11-epoxide levels resulting from an inhibition of epoxide hydrolase by valproate, without concurrent changes in plasma carbamazepine levels.

An AED may be the affected drug or the cause of an interaction. In fact, with some drug combinations, both the hepatic metabolism of the AED and that of the other drug are altered. For example, during co-medication with erythromycin and carbamazepine, carbamazepine plasma levels are elevated 2–4-fold due to inhibition of carbamazepine metabolism. Conversely, the effectiveness of standard dosages of erythromycin is reduced because carbamazepine enhances the metabolism of erythromycin. Other bi-directional interactions include those between topiramate and phenytoin, and between valproic acid and lamotrigine.

Introduction

Several drugs including macrolide antibiotics (e.g. erythromycin and troleandomycin) and hydrazines (e.g. isoniazid) undergo metabolic activation by CYP enzymes so that the formed metabolites bind to the prosthetic haem of CYPs to form stable metabolic intermediates rendering the CYP inactive. As CYP activity can only be restored by synthesis of new enzyme, the effect of such inhibitors may persist well after the elimination of the precursor (parent) drug. This mechanism is involved in the interaction between erythromycin and troleandomycin with carbamazepine (via inhibition of CYP3A4), and between isoniazid and phenytoin (via inhibition of CYP2C9).

Finally, inhibitory interactions can be irreversible in nature in that drugs containing certain functional groups can be oxidised by CYPs to reactive intermediates that subsequently cause irreversible inactivation of the CYP by alteration of haem or protein or a combination of both. An example of these "suicide inhibitors" is the furanocoumarins that are contained in grapefruit juice and irreversibly inhibit CYP3A4. Thus, grapefruit juice inhibits the metabolism of carbamazepine so that plasma carbamazepine levels are typically increased by 40%.

From a therapeutic viewpoint, drug interactions are best avoided by use of drugs that are not potent CYP inhibitors or inducers and are not readily inhibited by other drugs. In reality, drug interactions caused by mutual inhibition are almost inevitable, because CYP-mediated metabolism represents a major route of elimination of many drugs and because the same CYP enzymes can metabolise numerous drugs. The clinical significance of a metabolic drug interaction will depend on the magnitude of the change in the concentration of the active species (parent drug and/or metabolites) at the site of pharmacological action and the therapeutic index of the drug. The smaller the difference between toxicity and efficacy, the greater the likelihood that a drug interaction will have serious clinical consequences.

Anticipating and predicting metabolic interactions

In the past, drug interactions were identified essentially by serendipity. Typically, patients would complain of adverse effects or an increase in seizure frequency subsequent to the introduction of an additional drug to their drug regimen and upon investigation a drug interaction would be confirmed or refuted. In the late eighties formal drug interaction studies became an integral component of AED clinical trial development programmes but most drug interaction studies were conducted relatively late in Phase II and Phase III clinical development programmes and were based on a strategy that was in turn based on the therapeutic indices of drugs and the likelihood of their concurrent use. More recently, with the availability of human hepatic tissue and recombinant CYP enzymes, in vitro systems have been used as screening tools to predict the potential for in vivo drug interaction at a much earlier stage of drug development. The use of in vitro systems for investigating the ability of a drug to inhibit the metabolism of other drugs provides some of the most useful information in predicting potential drug-drug interactions. Nevertheless, the in vitro and clinical evaluation of all drugs with the potential to interact with an AED is not possible prior to licensing and thus interactions continue to come to light subsequent to licensing and during the drugs' availability for general clinical use.

In recent years our understanding of how individual drugs are metabolised has greatly facilitated the prediction of metabolic interactions. Whilst AEDs are metabolised in the liver via numerous pathways such as ß-oxidation (e.g. valproic acid) and conjugation involving UGTs (e.g. lamotrigine, oxcarbazepine and valproic acid), by far the most important system for AED metabolism is the CYP system (e.g. phenytoin, phenobarbital, carbamazepine, topiramate, tiagabine, zonisamide and felbamate). For an accurate prediction of a drug's potential to interact, it is essential to identify the enzyme(s) responsible for the metabolism of the drug. Furthermore, in order to be able to anticipate the possible clinical relevance of an interaction, it is important to determine the relative contribution of the metabolic pathway(s) being inhibited or induced to the overall elimination of the drug. In some cases, a single metabolic reaction may involve multiple isoforms or different enzyme systems, while in other cases all the metabolic reactions of a drug are catalysed by a single enzyme. The metabolism (S-oxidation) of 10-(N,N-dimethylaminoalkyl) phenothiazines is an example of the first scenario in which numerous CYP isoforms, including CYP2A6, CYP2C8 and CYP2D6, are involved in its metabolism. On the other hand the metabolism of indinavir, an HIV protease inhibitor, via four oxidative metabolic reactions (N-oxidation, N-dealkylation, indan hydroxylation and phenyl hydroxylation), is catalysed by a single isoform of CYP, namely CYP3A4.

Whilst *in vitro* data can be used to anticipate in vivo inhibitory interactions, such data are of very limited value is assessing the enzyme inducing properties of a

Introduction

drug. That the AEDs gabapentin, levetiracetam, pregabalin and vigabatrin do not undergo hepatic metabolism and neither inhibit nor induce CYP isoenzymes, provided a powerful predictor that these AEDs were unlikely to be associated with pharmacokinetic interactions and indeed this is the case clinically.

The clinical consequences of enzyme inhibition depend on the plasma level of the inhibitor, its inhibition constant for the enzyme, and the relative contribution of the pathway to the elimination of the affected drug. If the inhibited pathway accounts for only a small fraction (e.g. <30%-40%) of the drug's total clearance, the impact of the interaction on the drug's plasma level and clinical effect will be minimal. Age, genetics, and environmental factors may also influence the extent of inhibition. The effects of inhibition interactions are usually apparent within 24 hours of addition of the inhibitor, with time to the maximal increase in plasma levels determined by the time required for both the inhibitor and affected drug, which will now have a more prolonged half-life, to achieve steady-state. After discontinuation of the inhibitor, the time course for the decrease in plasma levels depends on the same factors.

In contrast to inhibitory interactions, interactions involving induction can be substantial even if induction involves a minor pathway of drug elimination. In this setting, the minor pathway may become the major pathway responsible for drug clearance causing a clinically relevant decrease in plasma levels.

Interactions with phenytoin, whereby the hepatic enzyme primarily responsible for the metabolism of phenytoin is the isoenzyme CYP2C9 (>80%) whilst CYP2C19 contributes <20% to the metabolism of phenytoin, need more thoughtful consideration. Thus, if amiodarone, fluconazole, miconazole, ketoconazole, propoxyphene or valproic acid (which inhibit CYP2C9), are co-administered with phenytoin they will have a substantial potential to inhibit phenytoin metabolism and elevate plasma phenytoin levels. In contrast, if topiramate, cimetidine, felbamate, omeprazole, fluoxetine or ticlopidine (which inhibit CYP2C19), are co-administered with phenytoin they will only have a small potential to inhibit phenytoin metabolism and elevate plasma phenytoin levels. However, while CYP2C19 is a minor pathway for phenytoin metabolism, its relative contribution increases at higher plasma levels due to saturation of the primary phenytoin pathway, CYP2C9. Thus, interactions with CYP2C19 inhibitors, while of minor importance at low phenytoin plasma levels, assume greater significance as plasma levels increase. Consequently, patients with phenytoin plasma levels above the saturable level for CYP2C9, which occur at or below the therapeutic range, are more prone to significant elevations in phenytoin plasma levels with the addition of CYP2C19 inhibitors.

Many interactions are associated with large inter-subject variability. In the case of interactions involving phenytoin, this can be explained by various factors. Firstly, there is significant inter-subject variability in the contribution of CYP2C9 and CYP2C19 to its metabolism. Secondly, it is known that drugs that inhibit CYP2C19 (without inhibiting CYP2C9), including carbamazepine, omeprazole, ticlopidine, felbamate and topiramate produce inconsistent elevations in phenytoin plasma levels. Thirdly, there is pharmacogenetic variability in CYP expression and a significant proportion of Caucasians and Asians exhibit the "poor metaboliser phenotype" of CYP2C19. In such subjects, inhibition of CYP2C19 is not manifested. Lastly, in the case of the interaction with carbamazepine, carbamazepine may increase the clearance of phenytoin through induction of CYP2C9 and/or CYP2C19.

A further confounding factor relates to the fact that drug interactions may relate to specific competitive inhibition of polymorphic enzymes. For example omeprazole and diazepam are predominantly metabolised by CYP2C19. The CYP2C19 isoform is known to be polymorphic and ~ 2-6% of Caucasians and 18-22% of Asians have been found to be poor metabolisers. Thus, patients that are extensive metabolisers of omeprazole, and consequently have a higher baseline metabolism of omeprazole, are more susceptible to enzyme inhibition interactions than are patients that are poor metabolisers of omeprazole. Similarly, extensive metabolisers are more susceptible to enzyme induction than poor metabolisers.

Databases listing substrates, inhibitors and inducers of different CYP isoenzymes provide an invaluable resource in helping the physician to predict and eventually to avoid potential interactions (Table 2). For example, knowledge that carbamazepine is an inducer of CYP3A4 allows one to predict that it will reduce the plasma level of CYP3A4 substrates such as ethosuximide, tiagabine, steroid oral contraceptives and cyclosporin. Likewise, the ability of ketoconazole to inhibit CYP3A4 explains the clinically important rise in plasma carbamazepine level after ingestion of this antifungal agent.

Introduction

Factors that impact on the relevance of a metabolic interaction

Although the number of theoretically possible interactions based on knowledge of the CYP and other enzyme systems (Table 2), are increasing, it must be appreciated that not all will be of clinical importance. The factors to be considered when evaluating the practical relevance of a potential interaction are as follows:

- The nature of the interaction at the enzyme site – is it a substrate, an inhibitor or an inducer?

- The spectrum of isoenzymes that are induced or inhibited by the interacting agent.

- The potency of the inhibition/induction – a potent effect will result in a more ubiquitous interaction affecting many/most patients.

- The concentration (level) of the inhibitor/inducer at the isoenzyme site – drugs that achieve low levels in blood may never reach the level threshold necessary to elicit an interaction.

- The extent of metabolism of the substrate through the particular isoenzyme – if the affected enzyme is only responsible for a small fraction of the drug's clearance, its inhibition is not going to result in a substantial interaction. Conversely, enzyme induction may increase the activity of the affected enzyme 7-fold, and therefore it may increase substantially the total clearance of the drug.

- The saturability of the isoenzyme – isoenzymes that are saturable at drug levels encountered clinically are more susceptible to significant inhibitory interactions.

- The route of administration – for drugs showing extensive first-pass metabolism, any change in plasma drug level caused by enzyme induction or inhibition will be much greater after oral than after parenteral administration.

- The presence of pharmacologically active metabolites – such metabolites complicate the outcome of a potential interaction, and may themselves act as enzyme inducers or inhibitors.

- The therapeutic window of the substrate – interactions affecting drugs with a narrow therapeutic window are more likely to be of clinical significance.

- The plasma level of the affected drug at baseline – any change in plasma drug

Table 2: Substrates, inhibitors and inducers of the major CYP isoenzymes involved in drug metabolism.
The list is intended for guidance only and should not be regarded as exhaustive. Prediction of drug interactions based on this Table should be with caution, because enzyme induction and inhibition may co-exist and because many other factors (see text) are involved in determining whether a clinically significant drug interaction will or will not occur.

Isoenzymes	Substrates	Inhibitors	Inducers
CYP1A2	**Psychotropic drugs:** Amitriptyline, clomipramine, chlorpromazine, clozapine, fluvoxamine, haloperidol, imipramine, mirtazapine, olanzapine **Miscellaneous:** Aminophylline, caffeine, dacarbazine, paracetamol, propranolol, sulindac, tacrine, tamoxifen, theophylline, verapamil, R-warfarin, zopiclone	**Non-AEDs:** Ciprofloxacin Clarithromycin Fluvoxamine Furafylline	**AEDs:** Carbamazepine Phenobarbital Phenytoin Primidone **Non-AEDs:** Charcoal-broiled meat Cigarette smoke Rifampicin Ritonavir St. John's wort
CYP2C9	**AEDs:** Phenobarbital, phenytoin, valproic acid **Non-steroidal antiinflammatory drugs:** Celecoxib, diclofenac, ibuprofen, naproxen, piroxicam **Psychotropic drugs:** Fluoxetine, olanzapine, quetiapine **Miscellaneous:** Amitriptyline, dicoumarol, fluvastatin, losartan, miconazole, phenylbutazone, theophylline, tolbutamide, torasemide, voriconazole, S-warfarin, zidovudine	**AEDs:** Valproic acid **Non-AEDs:** Amiodarone Chloramphenicol Delavirdine Efavirenz Fluconazole Fluoxetine Fluvoxamine Miconazole Sulfaphenazole Voriconazole	**AEDs:** Carbamazepine Phenobarbital Phenytoin Primidone **Non-AEDs:** Rifampicin Ritonavir St. John's wort
CYP2C19	**AEDs:** Diazepam, S-mephenytoin, methylphenobarbital, phenytoin **Psychotropic drugs:** Amitriptyline, citalopram, clomipramine, imipramine, moclobemide **Miscellaneous:** Lansoprazole, omeprazole, pantoprazole, proguanil, propranolol, voriconazole, R-warfarin	**AEDs:** Felbamate Oxcarbazepine Topiramate (weak) **Non-AEDs:** Cimetidine Delavirdine Efavirenz Esomeprazole Fluconazole Fluvoxamine Lansoprazole Omeprazole Ticlopidine	**AEDs:** Carbamazepine Phenobarbital Phenytoin Primidone **Non-AEDs:** Rifampicin Ritonavir

Isoenzymes	Substrates	Inhibitors	Inducers

CYP2D6

Psychotropic drugs: Amitriptyline, chlorpromazine, citalopram, clomipramine, clozapine, desipramine, fluoxetine, fluphenazine, fluvoxamine, haloperidol, imipramine, maprotiline, mianserin, mirtazapine, nefazodone, nortriptyline, olanzapine, paroxetine, perphenazine, quetiapine, risperidone, sertindole, thioridazine, venlafaxine, zuclopenthixol
Cardiovascular drugs: Alprenolol, bufuralol, encainide, flecainide, metoprolol, pindolol, propafenone, propranolol, timolol
Miscellaneous: Codeine, debrisoquine, dextromethorphan, phenformin, ritonavir, tamoxifen, tramadol

Inhibitors
Non-AEDs:
Cimetidine
Fluoxetine
Haloperidol
Lansoprazole
Paroxetine
Perphenazine
Propafenone
Quinidine
Terbinafine
Thioridazine

Inducers
No inducer known

CYP2E1

AEDs: Felbamate, phenobarbital
Miscellaneous: Chlorzoxazone, dapsone, ethanol, halothane, isoniazid

Non-AEDs:
Disulfiram

Non-AEDs:
Ethanol
Isoniazid

CYP3A4

AEDs: Carbamazepine, ethosuximide, tiagabine, zonisamide, some benzodiazepines (e.g., alprazolam, diazepam, midazolam, triazolam)
Psychotropic drugs: Amitriptyline, citalopram, clomipramine, clozapine, fluoxetine, fluvoxamine, haloperidol, imipramine, lercanidipine, mirtazapine, nefazodone, olanzapine, quetiapine, risperidone, sertindole, sertraline, trazodone, venlafaxine, ziprasidone
Cardiovascular drugs: Amiodarone, atorvastatin, diltiazem, felodipine, lacidipine, lovastatin, nifedipine, nimodipine, quinidine, simvastatin, verapamil
Chemotherapeutic drugs: Cyclophosphamide, dexamethasone, docetaxel, doxorubicin, etoposide, ifosfamide, irinotecan, paclitaxel, procarbazine, tamoxifen, teniposide, thiotepa, topotecan, vinblastine, vincristine, vindesine
Miscellaneous: Alfentanil, astemizole, cisapride, clarithromycin, cyclophosphamide, cyclosporin A, erythromycin, fentanyl, glucocorticoids, indinavir, isoniazid, itraconazole, ketoconazole, lidocaine, lopinavir, methadone, nefazodone, nevirapine, oral contraceptive, proguanil, quetiapine, rifampicin, ritonavir, saquinavir, sildenafil, steroids, tacrolimus, terfenadine, theophylline, troleandomycin, voriconazole

Inhibitors
Non-AEDs:
Amprenavir
Cimetidine
Clarithromycin
Cyclophosphamide
Cyclosporin A
Delavirdine
Dexamethasone
Dextropropoxyphene
Diltiazem
Docetaxel
Doxorubicin
Efavirenz
Erythromycin
Etoposide
Fluconazole
Fluoxetine
Fluvoxamine
Grapefruit juice
Ifosfamide
Indinavir
Isoniazid
Itraconazole
Ketoconazole
Lidocaine
Lopinavir
Methadone
Nefazodone
Nelfinavir
Nifedipine
Paclitaxel
Ritonavir
Teniposide
Troleandomycin
Venlafaxine
Verapamil
Vinblastine
Vindesine
Zidovudine

Inducers
AEDs:
Carbamazepine
Felbamate*
Oxcarbazepine*
Phenobarbital
Phenytoin
Primidone
Topiramate*

Non-AEDs:
Cyclophosphamide
Dexamethasone
Docetaxel
Efavirenz
Glucocorticoids*
Nefazodone
Nevirapine
Pacitaxel
Rifabutin
Rifampicin
St. John's wort
Tamoxifen
Teniposide

---

*These inducers are weaker or may induce CYP3A4 isoenzymes only in certain tissues

Only an inducer in females.

Figure 1: Strategies for managing interactions: dosage adjustments based on mechanism of drug interaction

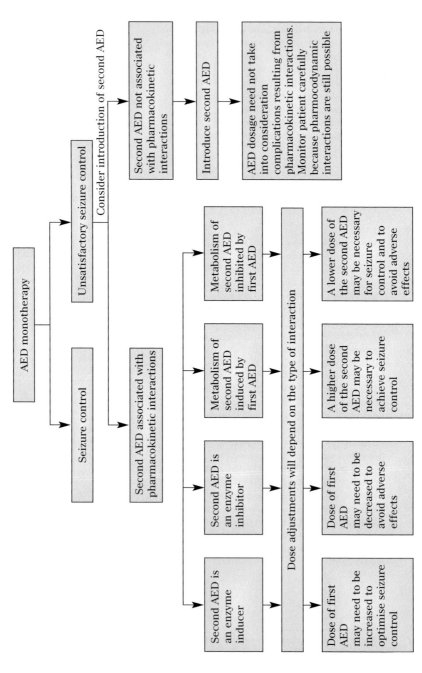

Reprinted with permission from Elsevier (The Lancet Neurology 2003;2:347-356) and the International League Against Epilepsy (Epilepsia 2002;43:365-385)

level will have greater consequences if the baseline level is near the threshold of toxicity (or near the threshold required to produce a desirable therapeutic effect).

- The genetic predisposition of the individual patient – for example, subjects who show deficiency of a genetically polymorphic isoenzyme (e.g., CYP2D6 or CYP2C19) will not exhibit interactions mediated by induction or inhibition of that isoenzyme.

- The susceptibility and the sensitivity of the individual in relation to adverse effects – the elderly are more susceptible to interactions because as a patient group they are more likely to receive multiple medications. Also the elderly are more sensitive to the adverse effects of drugs.

- The probability of the potential interacting drugs being co-prescribed – if a particular combination is unlikely to be co-prescribed, then any potential interaction will be of no clinical relevance.

Prevention and management of adverse AED interactions

Prevention of AED interactions is best achieved by avoiding unnecessary polytherapy or by selecting alternative agents that have less potential to interact. The management of interactions begins with anticipating their occurrence and being familiar with the mechanisms involved (Figure 1). Indeed, awareness of the mechanism of a drug interaction can be used to clinical advantage, for example, when one drug reduces the rate of elimination of another and increases the half-life of the affected drug; this can have an impact on the frequency of dosing, which in turn may improve compliance, or it may mean that a reduction of the dose of the affected drug is necessary. Also, in patients with a sub-therapeutic plasma level of drug, elevation of the level may actually result in better seizure control.

Introduction

By following a few simple rules, potential adverse consequences of AED interactions can be minimised or even avoided:

Rule 1:

Utilize multiple drug therapy only when it is clearly indicated. Most patients with epilepsy can be best managed with a carefully individualized dosage of a single AED.

Rule 2:

If a patient suffers from co-morbidities requiring multiple medications, it is preferable to treat the seizure disorder with an AED having a low interaction potential. Lamotrigine, topiramate, levetiracetam, tiagabine, gabapentin and pregabalin have little or no ability to cause enzyme induction or inhibition. Among AEDs, the lowest interaction potential is associated with the renaly eliminated agents gabapentin, levetiracetam, pregabalin and vigabatrin.

Rule 3:

Be aware of the most important interactions and their underlying mechanisms and any corrective action required (e.g. altered dosing requirements). Most interactions are metabolically based and can be predicted from knowledge of the isoenzymes responsible for the metabolism of the most commonly used drugs and the effects of these drugs on the same isoenzymes.

Rule 4:

Avoid combining AEDs with similar adverse effects profiles (e.g. benzodiazepines and barbiturates) or drugs associated with additive neurotoxicity (e.g. combinations of two sodium-channel blockers, such as carbamazepine and oxcarbazepine, or carbamazepine and lamotrigine are less well tolerated than combinations of drugs acting through different mechanisms) and select preferentially those combinations for which there is clinical evidence of favourable interactions (e.g. ethosuximide and valproate in refractory absence seizures or valproate and lamotrigine in the management of a wide variety of refractory seizures).

Rule 5:

Observe clinical response carefully whenever a drug is added or discontinued from the patient's regimen. Consider the possibility of an interaction if there is an unexpected change in response. Adjust dosage when appropriate.

Rule 6:

Be aware that some patient groups (e.g. the elderly, patients with renal or hepatic insufficiency and during pregnancy) may be more susceptible to interactions and/or more sensitive to the adverse effects of drugs. A contributing confounding factor amongst these patients is that their pharmacokinetic handling of drugs is altered.

Rule 7:

If a pharmacokinetic interaction is anticipated, monitor, if appropriate, the plasma level of the affected drug. Be aware that under certain circumstances (e.g. in the presence of drug displacement from plasma proteins), routine total drug level measurements may be misleading and patient management may benefit from monitoring of free non-protein bound drug levels (e.g. the interaction between valproic acid and phenytoin). In some cases, dosage adjustments may have to be implemented at the time the interacting drug is added or removed. Also, with some drugs, monitoring of surrogate therapeutic markers is preferable over blood level monitoring (e.g. with warfarin and dicoumarol it is advisable to monitor the INR [international normalized ratio] whenever a significant change in therapy of a concomitant enzyme inducing AED is made).

Rule 8:

When adding a drug to treat intercurrent or concomitant conditions, choose the one, which within a given class is least likely to be involved in worrisome problematic interactions. For example, famotidine would be preferable to cimetidine as an H_2 antagonist, and atenolol would be preferable to metoprolol as a ß-adrenoceptor blocker.

Rule 9:

Ask patients to report any symptoms or signs suggestive of overdosage or insufficient therapeutic cover.

Rule 10:

Inform patients of potential hazards associated with over-the-counter medicines, vitamin supplements and herbal products. Many such products are known to interfere with the metabolism of AEDs. Discuss in advance with patients and appropriate alternatives should be suggested e.g. cold or allergy preparations containing a sympathomimetic amine rather than antihistamines, non-alcoholic formulations of medications, and use of parenteral or oral nonsteroidal anti-inflammatory drugs rather than narcotic analgesics for mild-to-moderate pain control.

Figure 2: Strategies for managing interactions: dosage adjustments based on AED levels.

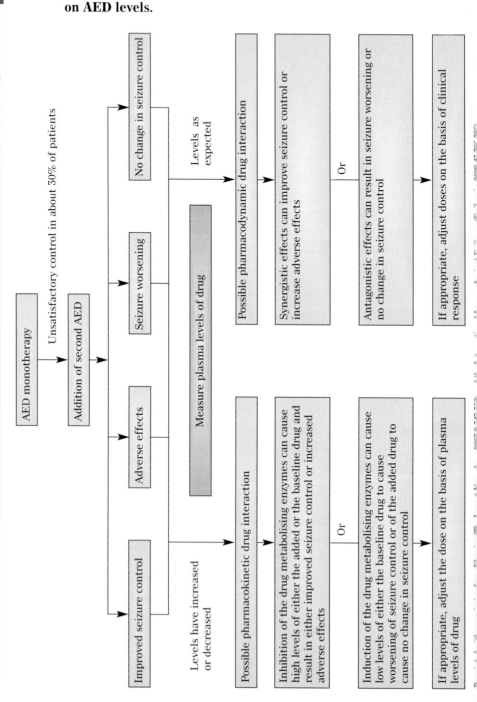

Introduction

The role of therapeutic drug monitoring in the management of AED interactions

Because AED interactions are primarily pharmacokinetic in nature, presenting with changes in drug plasma levels, it raises the question of the role for therapeutic drug monitoring in managing these interactions. For most AEDs there are well-accepted target ranges, however, this is not the case for non-AED drugs. Indeed, for many non-AED drugs there is still debate as to what would be the best parameter for measurement (trough [Cmin] or peak [Cmax] blood level or the area under the concentration versus time curve [AUC]). The best approach, in most clinical settings, is to undertake a drug level measurement before adding the new drug and then to use that value, as necessary, to adjust dosage to achieve the previously effective target level and response. It should be remembered, however, that for plasma protein binding displacement interactions, patient management may be best guided by the use of free (non-protein bound) plasma drug levels. *See figure 2 on previous page.*

With some drug interactions, surrogate markers other than plasma drug levels are better suited as a guide to clinical management. For example, it is advisable to monitor the INR (international normalized ratio) with warfarin and dicoumarol whenever a significant change in therapy of a concomitant enzyme inducing AED is made. Also, the determination of the viral load of HIV patients prescribed AEDs and antiviral medication may provide an invaluable indicator of an underlying interaction.

Generic and proprietary names of AEDs

Table 3 (overleaf)lists the generic names of all currently licensed antiepileptic drugs and also the proprietary names that are used world-wide.

Table 3: Antiepileptic drugs

Generic names	Proprietary names
Carbamazepine	Antafit, Atretol, Bioneuryl, Bioreunil, Carba, Carbabeta, Carbaflux, Carbagamma, Carbagen, Carbalan, Carbatrol, Carbaval, Carbazene, Carbazep, Carbazina, Carbi, Carbium Carmapine, Carpaz, Carpin, Carpine, Carzepine, Clostedal Degranol, Deleptin, Epimaz, Epitol, Espa-lepsin, Finlepsin Fitzecalm, Fokalepsin, Gericarb, Hermolepsin, Karbac, Mapezine, Neugeron, Neurotol, Neurotop, Nordotol, Novo-Carbamaz, Panitol, Sirtal, Taver, Tegretal, Tegretard, Tegretol, Temporol, Teril, Timonil, Trimonil, Voluto
Clobazam	Castilium, Frisium, Noiafen, Urbanil, Urbanol, Urbanyl
Clonazepam	Antelepsin, Clonapam, Clonex, Iktorivil, Kenoket, Klonipi Kriodex, Paxam, Rivatril, Rivotril
Ethosuximide	Emeside, Petinimid, Petridan, Suxilep, Suxinutin, Zarondan, Zarontin
Felbamate	Felbatol, Taloxa
Gabapentin	Aclonium, Equipax, Neurontin, Progresse
Lamotrigine	Labileno, Lamictin, Lamictal, Neurium
Levetiracetam	Keppra
Oxcarbazepine	Apydan, Auram, Trileptal, Trileptin
Phenobarbital (Phenobarbitone)	Adhanol, Alepsal, Aparoxal, Aphenylbarbit, Bialminal, Comizial, Fenemal, Fenocris, Gardenal, Gardenale, Gratusminal, Kaneuron, Lepinal, Lepinaletten, Lethyl, Luminal, Luminale, Luminaletas, Luminalette, Luminaletten, Neurobiol, Phenoemal, Phenoemaletten, Phenotal, Sudabarb, Sevium
Phenytoin (Diphenylhydantoin)	Aurantin, Dilantin, Dintoina, Diphantoin, Ditoin, Ditomed Di-Hydan, Epamin, Epanutin, Epelin, Epilan-D, Epilantine Epinat, Fenantoin, Fenidantal, Fenidantoin S, Fenital, Fenitron, Hidantal, Hidantina, Hidantoina, Hydantin, Lehydan, Neosidantoina, Nuctane, Pepsytoin, Phenhydan, Phenytek, Sinergina, Zentropil
Pregabalin	Lyrica
Primidone	Cyral, Liskantin, Mylepsinum, Mysoline, Prysoline, Resimat
Valproic acid (Sodium valproate)	Absenor, Atemperator, Convulex, Convulsofin, Criam, Delepsine, Depacan, Depakene, Depakin, Depakine, Depakote, Depalept, Depamog, Deprakine, Deproic, Diplexil, Encorate, Epiject, Epilenil, Epilim, Epival, Ergenyl, Leptilan, Leptilanil, Mylproin, Orfiril, Orlept, Pimiken, Valpakine, Valparin, Valporal, Valpra, Valprosid
Tiagabine	Gabatril, Gabitril
Topiramate	Epitomax, Topamax, Topimax
Vigabatrin	Sabril, Sabrilan, Sabrilex
Zonisamide	Zonegran

CARBAMAZEPINE

Metabolic profile

Biotransformation

Carbamazepine is extensively metabolised to carbamazepine-10,11-epoxide and then to carbamazepine-10,11-diol by cytochrome P450 enzymes. Whilst the formation of the epoxide is mediated primarily via CYP3A4, with some contribution by CYP2C8, the metabolism of the epoxide is via the enzyme epoxide hydrolase. Carbamazepine is an enzyme-inducer and its own metabolism is susceptible to autoinduction after repeated administration.

Renal excretion

Less than 2% of an administered dose is excreted unchanged in urine.

Pharmacokinetic characteristics

Elimination half-life of carbamazepine = **8-20 hours**

Elimination half-life of carbamazepine-10,11-epoxide = **6-15 hours**

New steady-state carbamazepine blood levels after inhibition of carbamazepine metabolism will occur **2-5 days later.**

New steady-state carbamazepine-10,11-epoxide blood levels after inhibition of carbamazepine-10,11-epoxide metabolism will occur **1.5-3 days later.**

Carbamazepine plasma protein binding = **70%**

Carbamazepine-10,11-epoxide plasma protein binding = **50%**

Therapeutic drug monitoring

Plasma target (therapeutic) level (concentration) for carbamazepine:
up to 50 μmol/L (12 μg/mL)

Plasma target (therapeutic) level (concentration) for carbamazepine10,11-epoxide:
up to 9 μmol/L (2.5 μg/mL)

Interactions with AEDs

Clonazepam:	Does not affect the pharmacokinetics of carbamazepine.
Ethosuximide:	Does not affect the pharmacokinetics of carbamazepine.
Felbamate:	Enhances the metabolism of carbamazepine.
Consequence:	Mean carbamazepine plasma levels can decrease by 30% and carbamazepine-10,11-epoxide levels (pharmacologically active metabolite of carbamazepine) increase by 57%. The interaction is the consequence of induction of carbamazepine metabolism through CYP3A4 and inhibition of the metabolism of carbamazepine-10,11-epoxide via an action on epoxide hydrolase.
Gabapentin:	Does not affect the pharmacokinetics of carbamazepine.
Lamotrigine	Does not affect the pharmacokinetics of carbamazepine.
Levetiracetam:	Does not affect the pharmacokinetics of carbamazepine.
	A pharmacodynamic interaction may occur whereby symptoms of carbamazepine toxicity present.
Oxcarbazepine:	Enhances the metabolism of carbamazepine.
Consequence:	Mean carbamazepine plasma levels can decrease by 13%. The interaction is the consequence of induction of carbamazepine metabolism through CYP3A4.
Phenobarbital:	Enhances the metabolism of carbamazepine.
Consequence:	Mean carbamazepine plasma levels can decrease by 33% and mean carbamazepine-10,11-epoxide levels (pharmacologically active metabolite of carbamazepine) increase by 24%. The interaction is the consequence of induction of carbamazepine metabolism through CYP3A4 and inhibition of the metabolism of carbamazepine-10,11-epoxide via an action on epoxide hydrolase.
Phenytoin:	Enhances the metabolism of carbamazepine.
Consequence:	Mean carbamazepine plasma levels can decrease by 44%. However, carbamazepine-10,11-epoxide levels (pharmacologically active metabolite of carbamazepine) are unaffected. The interaction is the consequence of induction of carbamazepine metabolism through CYP3A4.

Interactions with AEDs

Pregabalin:	Does not affect the pharmacokinetics of carbamazepine.
Primidone:	Enhances the metabolism of carbamazepine.
Consequence:	Mean carbamazepine plasma levels can decrease by 25% and mean carbamazepine-10,11-epoxide levels (pharmacologically active metabolite of carbamazepine) increase by 75%. The interaction is the consequence of induction of carbamazepine metabolism through CYP3A4 and inhibition of the metabolism of carbamazepine-10,11-epoxide via an action on epoxide hydrolase.
Tiagabine:	Does not affect the pharmacokinetics of carbamazepine.
Topiramate:	Does not affect the pharmacokinetics of carbamazepine.
Valproic acid:	Inhibits the metabolism of the pharmacologically active metabolite carbamazepine-10,11-epoxide.
Consequence:	Plasma levels of carbamazepine-10,11-epoxide (the active metabolite carbamazepine), with either no change or a small decrease in plasma carbamazepine levels, can increase by 2-fold. This interaction is related to valproic acid inhibition of epoxide hydrolase, the enzyme mediating the metabolism of the epoxide metabolite. Dosage adjustments should be primarily guided by clinical response but monitoring of carbamazepine-10,11-epoxide may serve to confirm the cause of adverse effects.
	During combination therapy, valproic acid synergistically enhances the antiepileptic efficacy (partial seizures) and toxicity of carbamazepine. These effects are probably the consequence of a pharmacodynamic interaction.
Vigabatrin:	Does not affect the pharmacokinetics of carbamazepine. There is a suggestion that in patients with low carbamazepine levels (<9 mg/mL) that plasma carbamazepine levels can be significantly elevated (20-132%), through an unknown mechanism, during concomitant administration with vigabatrin.
Zonisamide:	Inconsistent effect.
Consequence:	Reports are contradictory with plasma carbamazepine levels reported to both increase and decrease upon carbamazepine co-administration.

CLOBAZAM

Metabolic profile

Biotransformation

Clobazam is primarily metabolised by desmethylation to N-desmethylclobazam, but hydroxylation also occurs. The hydroxylation process results in the formation of other metabolites namely 4-hydroxyclobazam and 4-hydroxydesmethylclobazam. The N-desmethylclobazam metabolite is pharmacologically active and contributes significantly to the efficacy of clobazam.

Renal excretion

Renal excretion of unmetabolised clobazam is insignificant.

Pharmacokinetic characteristics

Elimination half-life of clobazam = **10-30 hours**

Elimination half-life of N-desmethylclobazam = **36-46 hours**

New steady-state clobazam blood levels after inhibition of clobazam metabolism will occur **2-8 days later.**

Clobazam plasma protein binding = **85%**

Therapeutic drug monitoring

Plasma target (therapeutic) level (concentration) for clobazam: **up to 670 μmol/L (200 μg/mL)**

Plasma target (therapeutic) level (concentration) for N-desmethylclobazam: **up to 7000 μmol/L (2000 μg/mL)**

Interactions with AEDs

Carbamazepine:	Enhances the metabolism of clobazam.
Consequence:	Plasma levels of the pharmacologically active metabolite of clobazam, N-desmethylclobazam, are increased during co-medication with carbamazepine. Typically the plasma level to weight-adjusted dose ratio of N-desmethylclobazam and clobazam can be expected to be 2-fold higher and 2-fold lower respectively.

Interactions with AEDs

Felbamate:	Inhibits the metabolism of clobazam.
Consequence:	Plasma levels of the pharmacologically active metabolite of clobazam, N-desmethylclobazam, are increased during co-medication with felbamate. Typically the plasma level to weight-adjusted dose ratio of N-desmethylclobazam and clobazam can be expected to be 5-fold higher and 2-fold lower respectively. The interaction may be the consequence of inhibition of N-desmethylclobazam metabolism through CYP2C19.
Lamotrigine:	Does not affect the pharmacokinetics of clobazam.
Levetiracetam:	Does not affect the pharmacokinetics of clobazam.
Phenobarbital:	Enhances the metabolism of clobazam.
Consequence:	Plasma levels of the pharmacologically active metabolite of clobazam, N-desmethylclobazam, are increased during co-medication with phenobarbital. Typically the plasma level to weight-adjusted dose ratio of N-desmethylclobazam and clobazam can be expected to be 2-fold higher and 2-fold lower respectively.
Phenytoin:	Enhances the metabolism of clobazam.
Consequence:	Plasma levels of the pharmacologically active metabolite of clobazam, N-desmethylclobazam, are increased during co-medication with phenytoin. Typically the plasma level to weight-adjusted dose ratio of N-desmethylclobazam and clobazam can be expected to be 2-fold higher and 2-fold lower respectively.
Primidone:	Primidone enhances the metabolism of clobazam.
Consequence:	Typically plasma levels of the pharmacologically active metabolite of clobazam, N-desmethylclobazam, are increased during co-medication with primidone. Typically the blood level to weight-adjusted dose ratio of N-desmethylclobazam and clobazam can be expected to be 2-fold higher and 2-fold lower respectively.

CLONAZEPAM

Metabolic profile

Biotransformation

Clonazepam is extensively metabolised by reduction (via CYP3A4) to produce 7-amino-clonazepam which is subsequently metabolised by acetylation (via N-acetyl-transferase) to form 7-acetamido-clonazepam. Clonazepam is also hydroxylated (isoenzyme not identified) to form 3-hydroxyclonazepam. None of the metabolites of clonazepam are pharmacologically active.

Renal excretion

Less than 1% of the dose of clonazepam is excreted unchanged in the urine.

Pharmacokinetic characteristics

Elimination half-life of clonazepam = **20-60 hours**

New steady-state clonazepam blood levels after inhibition of clonazepam metabolism will occur **4-15 days later**.

Plasma protein binding = **86%**

Therapeutic drug monitoring

Plasma target (therapeutic) level (concentration) for clonazepam: **up to 270 μmol/L (85 μg/mL)**

Interactions with AEDs

Carbamazepine: Enhances the metabolism of clonazepam.
Consequence: Plasma clonazepam levels can decrease by 19-37%.

Felbamate: Does not affect the pharmacokinetics of clonazepam.

Lamotrigine: Enhances the metabolism of clonazepam.
Consequence: Plasma clonazepam levels can decrease by <20-38%.

Phenobarbital: Enhances the metabolism of clonazepam.
Consequence: Plasma clonazepam levels can decrease by 19-24%.

Phenytoin: Enhances the metabolism of clonazepam.
Consequence: Plasma clonazepam levels can decrease by 46-58%.

ETHOSUXIMIDE

Metabolic profile

Biotransformation

Ethosuximide is eliminated primarily by metabolism with 30-60% of an administered dose recovered in urine as isomers of 2-(1-hydroxyethyl)-2-methylsuccinimide of which at least 40% are glucuronide conjugates. Metabolism is primarily mediated by CYP3A and to a lesser extent by CYP2E and CYP2B/C.

Renal excretion

Approximately 20% of an administered dose is excreted unchanged in urine.

Pharmacokinetic characteristics

Elimination half-life of ethosuximide = **40-60 hours**

New steady-state ethosuximide blood levels after inhibition of ethosuximide metabolism will occur **7-15 days later**.

Plasma protein binding = **0%**

Therapeutic drug monitoring

Plasma target (therapeutic) level (concentration) for ethosuximide: **up to 700 μmol/L (100 μg/mL)**

Interactions with AEDs

Carbamazepine:	Enhances the metabolism of ethosuximide.
Consequence:	The mean elimination half-life of ethosuximide can be decreased by 46% and clearance enhanced by 40% compared to ethosuximide monotherapy. The interaction is the consequence of induction of ethosuximide metabolism through CYP3A.
Felbamate:	The interaction has not been investigated. Theoretically a pharmacokinetic interaction could occur.
Gabapentin:	The interaction has not been investigated. Theoretically a pharmacokinetic interaction would not be anticipated.
Lamotrigine:	Does not affect the pharmacokinetics of ethosuximide.
Levetiracetam:	The interaction has not been investigated. Theoretically a pharmacokinetic interaction would not be anticipated.

Interactions with AEDs

Oxcarbazepine:	The interaction has not been investigated. Theoretically a pharmacokinetic interaction could occur.
Phenobarbital:	Enhances the metabolism of ethosuximide.
Consequence:	The mean elimination half-life of ethosuximide can be decreased by 46% and clearance enhanced by 40% compared to ethosuximide monotherapy. The interaction is the consequence of induction of ethosuximide metabolism through CYP3A.
Phenytoin:	Enhances the metabolism of ethosuximide.
Consequence:	The mean elimination half-life of ethosuximide can be decreased by 46% and clearance enhanced by 40% compared to ethosuximide monotherapy. The interaction is the consequence of induction of ethosuximide metabolism through CYP3A.
Pregabalin:	The interaction has not been investigated. Theoretically a pharmacokinetic interaction would not be anticipated.
Primidone:	Enhances the metabolism of ethosuximide.
Consequence:	The mean elimination half-life of ethosuximide can be decreased by 46% and clearance enhanced by 40% compared to ethosuximide monotherapy. The interaction is the consequence of induction of ethosuximide metabolism through CYP3A.
Primidone:	Enhances the metabolism of ethosuximide.
Consequence:	The mean elimination half-life of ethosuximide can be decreased by 46% and clearance enhanced by 40% compared to ethosuximide monotherapy. The interaction is the consequence of induction of ethosuximide metabolism through CYP3A.
Tiagabine:	The interaction has not been investigated. Theoretically a pharmacokinetic interaction would not be anticipated.
Topiramate:	The interaction has not been investigated. Theoretically a pharmacokinetic interaction would not be anticipated.

Drug Interactions Between AEDs

Interactions with AEDs

Valproic acid:	Reports are contradictory with plasma ethosuximide levels reported to decrease, increase and not change during co-administration with valproic acid.
Consequence:	The exact mechanisms involved are not known. Dosage adjustments may be necessary for some patients.
	During combination therapy, valproic acid synergistically enhances the antiepileptic efficacy (absence seizures) and toxicity of ethosuximide. These effects are probably the consequence of a pharmacodynamic interaction.
Vigabatrin:	The interaction has not been investigated. Theoretically a pharmacokinetic interaction would not be anticipated.
Zonisamide:	The interaction has not been investigated. Theoretically a pharmacokinetic interaction would not be anticipated.

FELBAMATE

Metabolic profile

Biotransformation

Only 50% of an administered dose is metabolised to form two hydroxylated metabolites (10-15% of metabolism) and a variety of other metabolites. None have significant pharmacological activity. The atroparaldehyde metabolite is hypothesised to be responsible or to contribute to the toxicity seen in some patients treated with felbamate. Felbamate is a substrate of CYP3A4 and CYP2E1.

Renal excretion

Approximately 40-50% of an absorbed dose is excreted unchanged in urine.

Pharmacokinetic characteristics

Elimination half-life of felbamate = **16-22 hours**

New steady-state felbamate blood levels after inhibition of felbamate metabolism will occur **3-6 days later**.

Plasma protein binding = **23%**

Therapeutic drug monitoring

Plasma target (therapeutic) level (concentration) for felbamate: up to **460 μmol/L (110 μg/mL)**

Interactions with AEDs

Carbamazepine:	Enhances the metabolism of felbamate.
Consequence:	The mean elimination half-life of felbamate can be decreased by 38% and clearance enhanced by 82%. The interaction is the consequence of induction of felbamate metabolism through CYP3A4.
Clonazepam:	Does not affect the pharmacokinetics of felbamate.
Ethosuximide:	The interaction has not been investigated. Theoretically a pharmacokinetic interaction would not be anticipated.

Interactions with AEDs

Gabapentin: The elimination of felbamate is reduced.

Consequence: The mean elimination half-life of felbamate can be reduced by 46% and clearance reduced by 37%. This interaction is considered to occur at the level of renal excretion.

Lamotrigine: Does not affect the pharmacokinetics of felbamate.

Levetiracetam: The interaction has not been investigated. Theoretically a pharmacokinetic interaction would not be anticipated.

Oxcarbazepine: Does not affect the pharmacokinetics of felbamate.

Phenobarbital: Enhances the metabolism of felbamate.

Consequence: The clearance of felbamate can be ~ 40% higher in patients receiving phenobarbital. The interaction is the consequence of induction of felbamate metabolism through CYP3A4.

Phenytoin: Enhances the metabolism of felbamate.

Consequence: Population pharmacokinetic studies report a 40% higher felbamate clearance in patients receiving phenytoin. The interaction is the consequence of induction of felbamate metabolism through CYP3A4.

Pregabalin: The interaction has not been investigated. Theoretically a pharmacokinetic interaction would not be anticipated.

Primidone: The interaction has not been investigated. Theoretically a pharmacokinetic interaction similar to that seen with phenobarbital can be expected.

Tiagabine: The interaction has not been investigated. Theoretically a pharmacokinetic interaction would not be anticipated.

Topiramate: The interaction has not been investigated. Theoretically a pharmacokinetic interaction could occur.

Valproic acid: Inhibits the metabolism of felbamate.

Consequence: The clearance of felbamate can be decreased by 13-21%.

Vigabatrin: Does not affect the pharmacokinetics of felbamate.

Zonisamide: The interaction has not been investigated. Theoretically a pharmacokinetic interaction could occur.

GABAPENTIN

Metabolic profile

Biotransformation

Gabapentin is not metabolised.

Renal excretion

Gabapentin is exclusively eliminated as unchanged gabapentin in urine.

Pharmacokinetic characteristics

Elimination half-life of gabapentin = **5-7 hours**

New steady-state gabapentin blood levels after inhibition of gabapentin elimination will occur **1-2 days later**.

Plasma protein binding = **0%**

Therapeutic drug monitoring

Plasma target (therapeutic) level (concentration) for gabapentin: up to **120 μmol/L (20 μg/mL)**

Interactions with AEDs

Carbamazepine:	Does not affect the pharmacokinetics of gabapentin.
Ethosuximide:	The interaction has not been investigated. Theoretically a pharmacokinetic interaction would not be anticipated.
Felbamate:	The interaction has not been investigated. Theoretically a pharmacokinetic interaction would not be anticipated.
Ethosuximide:	The interaction has not been investigated. Theoretically a pharmacokinetic interaction would not be anticipated.
Lamotrigine:	The interaction has not been investigated. Theoretically a pharmacokinetic interaction would not be anticipated.
Levetiracetam:	Does not affect the pharmacokinetics of gabapentin.
Oxcarbazepine:	The interaction has not been investigated. Theoretically a pharmacokinetic interaction would not be anticipated.
Phenobarbital:	Does not affect the pharmacokinetics of gabapentin.
Phenytoin:	Does not affect the pharmacokinetics of gabapentin.

Interactions with AEDs

Pregabalin:	The interaction has not been investigated. Because both pregabalin and gabapentin are absorbed via a common gastrointestinal uptake system, theoretically a pharmacokinetic interaction could occur whereby plasma gabapentin levels are reduced.
Primidone:	Does not affect the pharmacokinetics of gabapentin.
Tiagabine:	The interaction has not been investigated. Theoretically a pharmacokinetic interaction would not be anticipated.
Topiramate:	The interaction has not been investigated. Theoretically a pharmacokinetic interaction would not be anticipated.
Valproic acid:	Does not affect the pharmacokinetics of gabapentin.
Vigabatrin:	The interaction has not been investigated. Theoretically a pharmacokinetic interaction would not be anticipated.
Zonisamide:	The interaction has not been investigated. Theoretically a pharmacokinetic interaction would not be anticipated.

LAMOTRIGINE

Metabolic profile

Biotransformation

Lamotrigine undergoes extensive metabolism via glucuronidation and the primary metabolite is N-2 glucuronide (71% of dose). The metabolite N-5 glucuronide represents only 9% of metabolised lamotrigine. Glucuronidation is a major conjugation reaction that is catalysed by a number of different isoforms of UDP-glucuronosyltransferase (UGT). The N-2 glucuronidation of lamotrigine is catalysed by UGT1A4.

Renal excretion

Approximately 10% of administered lamotrigine is excreted unchanged in urine.

Pharmacokinetic characteristics

Elimination half-life of lamotrigine = **8-33 hours**

New steady-state lamotrigine blood levels after inhibition of lamotrigine metabolism will occur **2-9 days later**.

Plasma protein binding = **50%**

Therapeutic drug monitoring

Plasma target (therapeutic) level (concentration) for lamotrigine: **up to 60 μmol/L (15 μg/mL)**

Interactions with AEDs

Carbamazepine: Enhances the metabolism of lamotrigine.

Consequence: Mean plasma lamotrigine levels can be decreased by 52%. As a result, lamotrigine therapy is started at a higher dose and maintenance dose requirements are generally 2-4-fold higher in patients receiving carbamazepine compared to lamotrigine monotherapy. The interaction is the consequence of induction of lamotrigine metabolism through UGT1A4 glucuronidation.

The high frequency of neurotoxicity observed with this drug combination represents a pharmacodynamic rather than pharmacokinetic interaction.

Interactions with AEDs

Clonazepam:	The interaction has not been investigated. However, the in vitro metabolism of lamotrigine is minimally affected by clonazepam.
Ethosuximide:	The interaction has not been investigated. Theoretically a pharmacokinetic interaction would not be anticipated.
Felbamate:	Does not affect the pharmacokinetics of lamotrigine.
Gabapentin:	The interaction has not been investigated. Theoretically a pharmacokinetic interaction would not be anticipated.
Levetiracetam:	Does not affect the pharmacokinetics of lamotrigine.
Methsuximide:	Enhances the metabolism of lamotrigine.
Consequence:	Mean plasma lamotrigine levels can be decrease by 60%. The interaction is the consequence of induction of lamotrigine metabolism through UGT1A4 glucuronidation.
Oxcarbazepine:	Enhances the metabolism of lamotrigine.
Consequence:	Mean plasma lamotrigine levels can be decreased by 34%. The interaction is the consequence of induction of lamotrigine metabolism probably through UGT1A4 glucuronidation.
Phenobarbital:	Enhances the metabolism of lamotrigine.
Consequence:	Mean plasma lamotrigine levels can be decreased by 39%. As a result, lamotrigine therapy is started at a higher dose and maintenance dose requirements are generally 2-4-fold higher in patients receiving phenobarbital compared to lamotrigine monotherapy. The interaction is the consequence of induction of lamotrigine metabolism through UGT1A4 glucuronidation.
Phenytoin:	Enhances the metabolism of lamotrigine.
Consequence:	Mean plasma lamotrigine levels can be decreased by 48%. As a result, lamotrigine therapy is started at a higher dose and maintenance dose requirements are generally 2-4-fold higher in patients receiving phenytoin compared to lamotrigine monotherapy. The interaction is the consequence of induction of lamotrigine metabolism through UGT1A4 glucuronidation.
Pregabalin:	Does not affect the pharmacokinetics of lamotrigine.

Interactions with AEDs

Primidone:	The interaction has not been investigated. Theoretically an interaction similar to that seen with phenobarbital can be expected.
Tiagabine:	The interaction has not been investigated. Theoretically a pharmacokinetic interaction would not be anticipated.
Topiramate:	Does not affect the pharmacokinetics of lamotrigine.
Valproic acid:	Inhibits the metabolism of lamotrigine.
Consequence:	Mean plasma lamotrigine levels can be increased 2-fold. As a result, patients receiving this combination generally require less than one-half the dose of patients receiving lamotrigine monotherapy. The interaction is the consequence of inhibition of lamotrigine metabolism through UGT1A4 glucuronidation.

Concurrent valproic acid therapy is a risk factor for the development of skin rash with lamotrigine. The introduction of lamotrigine to patients already taking valproic acid should be undertaken with caution, using a low starting dose and a slow dose escalation rate. However, there is no risk of rash if valproic acid is introduced to patients already stabilised on lamotrigine.

During combination therapy, valproic acid synergistically enhances the antiepileptic efficacy (partial and generalised seizures) and toxicity of lamotrigine. This is considered to be the consequence of a pharmacodynamic interaction.

Vigabatrin:	The interaction has not been investigated. Theoretically a pharmacokinetic interaction would not be anticipated.
Zonisamide:	Does not affect the pharmacokinetics of lamotrigine.

LEVETIRACETAM

Metabolic profile

Biotransformation

Levetiracetam undergoes minimal metabolism with approximately 30% being metabolised (hydrolysis) non-hepatically in blood to an inactive metabolite.

Renal excretion

The elimination of levetiracetam is predominant renal with approximately 70% of a levetiracetam dose excreted unchanged in urine.

Pharmacokinetic characteristics

Elimination half-life of levetiracetam = 5-11 hours

New steady-state levetiracetam blood levels after inhibition of levetiracetam elimination will occur **1-3 days later.**

Plasma protein binding = **0%**

Therapeutic drug monitoring

Plasma target (therapeutic) level (concentration) for levetiracetam: **up to 120 mmol/L (20 mg/mL)**

Interactions with AEDs

Carbamazepine: Does not affect the pharmacokinetics of levetiracetam.

Clobazam: Does not affect the pharmacokinetics of levetiracetam.

Ethosuximide: The interaction has not been investigated. Theoretically a pharmacokinetic interaction would not be anticipated.

Felbamate: The interaction has not been investigated. Theoretically a pharmacokinetic interaction would not be anticipated.

Gabapentin: Does not affect the pharmacokinetics of levetiracetam.

Lamotrigine: Does not affect the pharmacokinetics of levetiracetam.

Interactions with AEDs

Oxcarbazepine: The interaction has not been investigated. Theoretically a pharmacokinetic interaction would not be anticipated.

Phenobarbital: Does not affect the pharmacokinetics of levetiracetam.

Phenytoin: Does not affect the pharmacokinetics of levetiracetam.

Pregabalin: Does not affect the pharmacokinetics of levetiracetam.

Primidone: Does not affect the pharmacokinetics of levetiracetam.

Tiagabine: The interaction has not been investigated. Theoretically a pharmacokinetic interaction would not be anticipated.

Topiramate: The interaction has not been investigated. Theoretically a pharmacokinetic interaction would not be anticipated.

Valproic acid: Does not affect the pharmacokinetics of levetiracetam.

Vigabatrin: The interaction has not been investigated. Theoretically a pharmacokinetic interaction would not be anticipated.

Zonisamide: The interaction has not been investigated. Theoretically a pharmacokinetic interaction would not be anticipated.

OXCARBAZEPINE

Metabolic profile

Biotransformation

Oxcarbazepine undergoes rapid and extensive metabolism to its pharmacologically active metabolite, 10-hydroxycarbazepine, by stereoselective biotransformation mediated by a cytosolic, non-microsomal, and non-inducible arylketone reductase. 10-hydroxycarbazepine is subsequently eliminated by glucuronidation (51%) or undergoes hydroxylation to form a dihydrodiol metabolite (28%). Only the latter reaction depends on CYP isoenzymes.

Renal excretion

Only <1% of oxcarbazepine is excreted unchanged in urine.

Pharmacokinetic characteristics

Elimination half-life of 10-hydroxycarbazepine = **8-15 hours**

New steady-state 10-hydroxycarbazepine blood levels after inhibition of 10-hydroxycarbazepine metabolism will occur **2-4 days later**.

Plasma protein binding of 10-hydroxycarbazepine = **40%**

Therapeutic drug monitoring

Plasma target (therapeutic) level (concentration) for 10-hydroxycarbazepine: up to **110 μmol/L (28 μg/mL)**

During treatment with oxcarbazepine only the pharmacologically active metabolite, 10-hydroxycarbazepine, is monitored because oxcarbazepine is very rapidly metabolised to its metabolite and therefore oxcarbazepine is essentially not detectable in blood by 1 hour post-ingestion.

Interactions with AEDs

Carbamazepine:	Enhances the metabolism of 10-hydroxycarbazepine.
Consequence:	The mean AUC value for 10-hydroxycarbazepine can be decreased by 40%. The mean elimination half-life of 10-hydroxycarbazepine can be decreased by 15%.
Clobazam:	Does not affect the pharmacokinetics of 10-hydroxycarbazepine.
Ethosuximide:	The interaction has not been investigated. Theoretically a pharmacokinetic interaction would not be anticipated.

Interactions with AEDs

Felbamate:	Does not affect the pharmacokinetics of 10-hydroxycarbazepine.
Gabapentin:	The interaction has not been investigated. Theoretically a pharmacokinetic interaction would not be anticipated.
Lamotrigine:	The interaction has not been investigated. Theoretically a pharmacokinetic interaction would not be anticipated.
Levetiracetam:	The interaction has not been investigated. Theoretically a pharmacokinetic interaction would not be anticipated.
Phenobarbital:	Enhances the metabolism of 10-hydroxycarbazepine.
Consequence:	The mean elimination half-life of 10-hydroxycarbazepine can be decreased by 15%.
Phenytoin:	Enhances the metabolism of 10-hydroxycarbazepine.
Consequence:	The mean AUC value for 10-hydroxycarbazepine can be decreased by 29%.
Pregabalin:	The interaction has not been investigated. Theoretically a pharmacokinetic interaction would not be anticipated.
Primidone:	The interaction has not been investigated. Theoretically an interaction similar to that seen with phenobarbital can be expected.
Tiagabine:	The interaction has not been investigated. Theoretically a pharmacokinetic interaction would not be anticipated.
Topiramate:	The interaction has not been investigated. Theoretically a pharmacokinetic interaction would not be anticipated.
Valproic acid:	Valproic acid displaces 10-hydroxycarbazepine from its plasma protein binding sites.
Consequence:	During combination therapy with valproic acid, 10-hydroxycarbazepine binding is 36% versus 47% for monotherapy oxcarbazepine. Clinical management may best be guided by monitoring free blood levels of 10-hydroxycarbazepine.
Vigabatrin:	The interaction has not been investigated. Theoretically a pharmacokinetic interaction would not be anticipated.
Zonisamide:	The interaction has not been investigated. Theoretically a pharmacokinetic interaction could occur.

PHENOBARBITAL

Metabolic profile

Biotransformation

Phenobarbital is extensively metabolised to two major metabolites, p-hydroxyphenobarbital, which partially undergoes sequential metabolism to a glucuronic acid conjugate, and 9-D-glucopyranosylphenobarbital, an N-glucoside conjugate (PNG). CYP2C9 plays a major role in the metabolism of phenobarbital to p-hydroxyphenobarbital with minor metabolism by CYP2C19 and CYP2E1. The identity of the UGT enzyme that is responsible for the formation of PNG is unknown. Phenobarbital is an enzyme-inducer.

Renal excretion

Approximately 25% of phenobarbital is eliminated as unchanged phenobarbital in urine.

Pharmacokinetic characteristics

Elimination half-life of phenobarbital = **50-160 hours**

New steady-state phenobarbital blood levels after inhibition of phenobarbital metabolism will occur **9-40 days later**.

Plasma protein binding = **50%**

Therapeutic drug monitoring

Plasma target (therapeutic) level (concentration) for phenobarbital: up to **170 μmol/L (40 μg/mL)**

Interactions with AEDs

Carbamazepine:	Does not affect the pharmacokinetics of phenobarbital.
Clonazepam:	Does not affect the pharmacokinetics of phenobarbital.
Ethosuximide:	Does not affect the pharmacokinetics of phenobarbital.
Felbamate:	Inhibits the metabolism of phenobarbital.
Consequence:	Plasma phenobarbital levels can be increased by 20-25%. The interaction is the consequence of inhibition of phenobarbital metabolism through CYP2C19.
Gabapentin:	Does not affect the pharmacokinetics of phenobarbital.

Interactions with AEDs

Lamotrigine:	Does not affect the pharmacokinetics of phenobarbital.
Levetiracetam:	Does not affect the pharmacokinetics of phenobarbital.
Oxcarbazepine:	Inhibits the metabolism of phenobarbital.
Consequence:	At oxcarbazepine dosages above 1200 mg/day, mean plasma phenobarbital levels can be increased by 15%. The interaction is the consequence of inhibition of phenobarbital metabolism through CYP2C19.
Phenytoin:	Inhibits the metabolism of phenobarbital.
Consequence:	Plasma phenobarbital levels can be increased by 50-70%. The interaction is the consequence of inhibition of phenobarbital metabolism through CYP2C19.
Pregabalin:	Does not affect the pharmacokinetics of phenobarbital.
Primidone:	Not commonly co-prescribed.
Tiagabine:	Does not affect the pharmacokinetics of phenobarbital.
Topiramate:	Does not affect the pharmacokinetics of phenobarbital.
Valproic acid:	Inhibits the metabolism of phenobarbital.
Consequence:	The extent of this interaction is characterised by considerable inter-individual variability with 50-80% of patients requiring a reduction in phenobarbital dose. Increases in mean plasma phenobarbital levels are greater in children (112%) compared to adults (51%).
Vigabatrin:	Does not affect the pharmacokinetics of phenobarbital.
Zonisamide:	Does not affect the pharmacokinetics of phenobarbital.

PHENYTOIN

Metabolic profile

Biotransformation

Phenytoin is eliminated almost entirely by metabolic transformation. The principal metabolites are p-hydroxyphenytoin (67-88%) and a dihydrodiol (7-11%). The first step in this pathway is the formation of an arene oxide intermediate through the isoenzymes CYP2C9 and CYP2C19. The arene oxide is converted spontaneously to form p-hydroxyphenytoin and is converted by the enzyme epoxide hydrolase to dihydrodiol. Phenytoin is an enzyme-inducer.

Renal excretion

Less than 5% of an administered phenytoin dose is excreted unchanged in urine.

Pharmacokinetic characteristics

Elimination half-life of phenytoin = **7-60 hours**

New steady-state phenytoin blood levels after inhibition of phenytoin metabolism will occur **2-15 days later.**

Plasma protein binding = **92%**

Therapeutic drug monitoring

Plasma target (therapeutic) level (concentration) for phenytoin: up to **80 μmol/L (20 μg/mL)**

Interactions with AEDs

Carbamazepine:	Conflicting results are observed.
Consequence:	Plasma phenytoin levels may decrease, remain the same, or increase after addition of carbamazepine. This is a consequence of inter-subject variability in CYP isoenzyme expression of CYP2C19 which carbamazepine inhibits and the fact that carbamazepine may increase the clearance of phenytoin through induction of CYP2C9 and/or CYP2C19.
Clobazam:	Inhibits the metabolism of phenytoin.
Consequence:	Plasma phenytoin levels can be increased by 25 - 75%.
Clonazepam:	Does not affect the pharmacokinetics of phenytoin.

Interactions with AEDs

Ethosuximide:	Does not affect the pharmacokinetics of phenytoin.
Felbamate:	Inhibits the metabolism of phenytoin.
Consequence:	Mean plasma phenytoin levels can be increased by ~ 30% and ~ 100% at 1,200 and 2,400 mg/day felbamate respectively. The interaction is the consequence of inhibition of phenytoin metabolism through CYP2C19.
Gabapentin:	Does not affect the pharmacokinetics of phenytoin.
Lamotrigine:	Does not affect the pharmacokinetics of phenytoin.
Levetiracetam:	Does not affect the pharmacokinetics of phenytoin.
Oxcarbazepine:	Inhibits the metabolism of phenytoin.
Consequence:	At oxcarbazepine dosages above 1200 mg/day, mean plasma phenytoin levels can be increased by 40%. The interaction is the consequence of inhibition of phenytoin metabolism through CYP2C19.
Phenobarbital	Conflicting results are observed.
Consequence:	Plasma phenytoin levels have been reported to increase, decrease, or not change upon the addition of phenobarbital. This variability reflects the fact that phenobarbital is both a CYP enzyme inducer and an inhibitor (substrate). In most patients, only small changes in blood levels occur and no dosage modification is needed. However, because of variability in the magnitude and direction of the interaction, clinical response and plasma phenytoin levels should be monitored.
Pregabalin:	Does not affect the pharmacokinetics of phenytoin.
Primidone:	The interaction has not been extensively investigated.
Consequence:	As primidone is metabolised to phenobarbital, the interaction profile described under phenobarbital can be expected to similarly occur for primidone.
Tiagabine:	Does not affect the pharmacokinetics of phenytoin.

Interactions with AEDs

Topiramate: Inhibits the metabolism of phenytoin.

Consequence: The magnitude of the interaction is variable with plasma phenytoin levels increasing by up to 25%. The interaction is the consequence of inhibition of phenytoin metabolism through CYP2C19.

Valproic acid: Conflicting results are observed.

Consequence: The effect of valproic acid on plasma phenytoin levels varies amongst patients and may vary in the same patient during the course of therapy. Thus, a persistent fall, a transient fall or even a rise can occur is some patients. These effects are the consequence of a displacement of phenytoin from its plasma protein (albumin) binding sites and the concurrent inhibition of CYP2C9 metabolism. The free fraction of phenytoin is increased. Clinically, the need to adjust phenytoin dosage is rare but if adjustment is necessary, it might best be guided by measurement of free (non-protein bound) phenytoin levels.

Vigabatrin: Plasma phenytoin levels are reduced.

Consequence: During co-medication with vigabatrin plasma phenytoin levels can decrease by up to 40%. The mechanism of this interaction is not known but does not involve any absorption or metabolic processes.

Zonisamide: Inhibits the metabolism of phenytoin.

Consequence: Population pharmacokinetic analysis shows a 16% increase in plasma phenytoin levels. The interaction is the consequence of inhibition of phenytoin metabolism through CYP2C19.

PREGABALIN

Metabolic profile

Biotransformation

Pregabalin is not metabolised.

Renal excretion

Pregabalin is exclusively eliminated as unchanged pregabalin in urine.

Pharmacokinetic characteristics

Elimination half-life of pregabalin = **5-7 hours.**

New steady-state pregabalin blood levels after inhibition of pregabalin elimination will occur **1-2 days later.**

Plasma protein binding = **0%**

Therapeutic drug monitoring

Plasma target (therapeutic) level (concentration) for pregabalin: **recommendations are not yet available.**

Interactions with AEDs

Carbamazepine:	Does not affect the pharmacokinetics of pregabalin.
Ethosuximide:	The interaction has not been investigated. Theoretically a pharmacokinetic interaction would not be anticipated.
Felbamate:	The interaction has not been investigated. Theoretically a pharmacokinetic interaction would not be anticipated.
Gabapentin:	The interaction has not been investigated. Because both pregabalin and gabapentin are absorbed via a common gastrointestinal uptake system, theoretically a pharmacokinetic interaction could occur whereby plasma pregabalin levels are reduced.
Lamotrigine:	Does not affect the pharmacokinetics of pregabalin.
Levetiracetam:	Does not affect the pharmacokinetics of pregabalin.
Oxcarbazepine:	The interaction has not been investigated. Theoretically a pharmacokinetic interaction would not be anticipated.
Phenobarbital:	Does not affect the pharmacokinetics of pregabalin.

Interactions with AEDs

Phenytoin:	Does not affect the pharmacokinetics of pregabalin.
Primidone:	The interaction has not been investigated. Theoretically a pharmacokinetic interaction would not be anticipated.
Tiagabine:	Does not affect the pharmacokinetics of pregabalin.
Topiramate:	Does not affect the pharmacokinetics of pregabalin.
Valproic acid:	Does not affect the pharmacokinetics of pregabalin.
Vigabatrin:	The interaction has not been investigated. Theoretically a pharmacokinetic interaction would not be anticipated.
Zonisamide:	The interaction has not been investigated. Theoretically a pharmacokinetic interaction would not be anticipated.

PRIMIDONE

Metabolic profile

Biotransformation

Primidone is metabolised to two pharmacologically active metabolites, namely phenylethylmalonamide and phenobarbital. The primary metabolite, phenobarbital, subsequently undergoes oxidation to form p-hydroxyphenobarbital. Primidone, via its metabolite phenobarbital, is an enzyme-inducer.

Renal excretion

During monotherapy, approximately 65% of primidone is excreted unchanged in urine. In contrast, during polytherapy with other hepatic enzyme-inducing antiepileptic drugs only 40% is excreted in urine as unchanged primidone.

Pharmacokinetic characteristics

Elimination half-life of primidone = **4-12 hours**.

New steady-state primidone blood levels after inhibition of primidone metabolism will occur **1-3 days later**.

Plasma protein binding = **15%**

Therapeutic drug monitoring

Plasma target (therapeutic) level (concentration) for primidone:
up to 60 μmol/L (13 μg/mL)

Plasma target (therapeutic) level (concentration) for phenobarbital: up to
170 μmol/L (40 μg/mL)

Interactions with AEDs

Carbamazepine: Enhances the metabolism of primidone.

Consequence: In patients receiving primidone, carbamazepine may cause a decrease in primidone and an increase in phenobarbital plasma levels.

Clobazam: Inhibits the metabolism of primidone.

Consequence: In children receiving primidone, clobazam decreases the clearance of primidone so that plasma primidone levels are increased.

Interactions with AEDs

Ethosuximide: The interaction has not been investigated. Theoretically a pharmacokinetic interaction would not be anticipated.

Felbamate: The interaction has not been investigated. Theoretically a pharmacokinetic interaction could occur.

Gabapentin: The interaction has not been investigated. Theoretically a pharmacokinetic interaction would not be anticipated.

Lamotrigine: Does not affect the pharmacokinetics of primidone.

Levetiracetam: Does not affect the pharmacokinetics of primidone.

Oxcarbazepine: The interaction has not been investigated. Theoretically a pharmacokinetic interaction could occur.

Phenobarbital: Combination not commonly co-prescribed.

Phenytoin: Enhances the metabolism of primidone.

Consequence: Phenytoin may cause a 10-30% decrease in plasma primidone levels and a 2-3-fold increase in plasma phenobarbital levels.

Pregabalin: The interaction has not been investigated. Theoretically a pharmacokinetic interaction would not be anticipated.

Tiagabine: Does not affect the pharmacokinetics of primidone.

Topiramate: Does not affect the pharmacokinetics of primidone.

Valproic acid: The metabolism of primidone to phenobarbital is unaffected but the subsequent metabolism of phenobarbital is inhibited.

Consequence: Mean plasma phenobarbital levels can increase by 51%. Plasma primidone levels are unaffected.

Vigabatrin: Does not affect the pharmacokinetics of primidone.

Zonisamide: Does not affect the pharmacokinetics of primidone.

TIAGABINE

Metabolic profile

Biotransformation

Tiagabine is extensively metabolised to two 5-oxo-tiagabine isomers by CYP3A-mediated activity.

Renal excretion

Only 2% of tiagabine is excreted in the unchanged form in urine.

Pharmacokinetic characteristics

Elimination half-life of tiagabine = **4-9 hours**

New steady-state tiagabine blood levels after inhibition of tiagabine metabolism will occur **1-3 days later**.

Plasma protein binding = **96%**

Therapeutic drug monitoring

Plasma target (therapeutic) level (concentration) for tiagabine: up to **1100 μmol/L (415 μg/mL)**

Interactions with AEDs

Carbamazepine: Enhances the metabolism of tiagabine.

Consequence: The elimination half-life of tiagabine in patients taking carbamazepine (plus other enzyme inducing AEDs) is 3.8-4.9 hours compared to 5-8 hours in healthy volunteers. Mean plasma tiagabine levels can be expected to be decreased by 40-70%. The interaction is the consequence of induction of tiagabine metabolism through CYP3A4.

Ethosuximide: The interaction has not been investigated. Theoretically a pharmacokinetic interaction would not be anticipated.

Felbamate: The interaction has not been investigated. Theoretically a pharmacokinetic interaction could occur.

Gabapentin: The interaction has not been investigated. Theoretically a pharmacokinetic interaction would not be anticipated.

Lamotrigine: The interaction has not been investigated. Theoretically a pharmacokinetic interaction would not be anticipated.

Interactions with AEDs

Levetiracetam: The interaction has not been investigated. Theoretically a pharmacokinetic interaction would not be anticipated.

Oxcarbazepine: The interaction has not been investigated. Theoretically a pharmacokinetic interaction could occur.

Phenobarbital: Enhances the metabolism of tiagabine.

Consequence: The elimination half-life of tiagabine in patients taking phenobarbital (plus other enzyme inducing AEDs) is 3.8-4.9 hours compared to 5-8 hours in healthy volunteers. Mean plasma tiagabine levels can be expected to be decreased by 40-70%. The interaction is the consequence of induction of tiagabine metabolism through CYP3A4.

Pregabalin: Does not affect the pharmacokinetics of tiagabine.

Phenytoin: Enhances the metabolism of tiagabine.

Consequence: The elimination half-life of tiagabine in patients taking phenytoin (plus other enzyme inducing AEDs) is 3.8-4.9 hours compared to 5-8 hours in healthy volunteers. Mean plasma tiagabine levels can be expected to be decreased by 40-70%. The interaction is the consequence of induction of tiagabine metabolism through CYP3A4.

Primidone: Enhances the metabolism of tiagabine.

Consequence: The elimination half-life of tiagabine patients taking primidone (plus other enzyme inducing AEDs) is 3.8-4.9 hours compared to 5-8 hours in healthy volunteers. Mean plasma tiagabine levels can be expected to be decreased by 40-70%. The interaction is the consequence of induction of tiagabine metabolism through CYP3A4.

Topiramate: The interaction has not been investigated. Theoretically a pharmacokinetic interaction could occur.

Valproic acid: Does not affect the pharmacokinetics of tiagabine.

Vigabatrin: The interaction has not been investigated. Theoretically a pharmacokinetic interaction would not be anticipated.

Zonisamide: The interaction has not been investigated. Theoretically a pharmacokinetic interaction would not be anticipated.

TOPIRAMATE

Metabolic profile
Biotransformation

In the absence of hepatic enzyme inducers, only 40% of topiramate is metabolised, whilst in the presence of hepatic enzyme inducers this value is doubled. Metabolites thus far identified include two hydroxy and two diol metabolites as well as several glucuronide conjugates. Although the specific CYP isoenzymes responsible for the metabolism of topiramate have not been identified, it is evident that isoenzymes induced by carbamazepine and phenytoin play a major role.

Renal excretion

Approximately 20-60% of topiramate is excreted in urine as unchanged topiramate.

Pharmacokinetic characteristics

Elimination half-life of topiramate = **12-30 hours**

New steady-state topiramate blood levels after inhibition of topiramate metabolism will occur **2-8 days later**.

Plasma protein binding = **10%**

Therapeutic drug monitoring

Plasma target (therapeutic) level (concentration) for topiramate: **up to 74 μmol/L (25 μg/mL)**

Interactions with AEDs

Carbamazepine: Enhances the metabolism of topiramate.
Consequence: Plasma topiramate levels can be decreased by up to 68%.

Ethosuximide: The interaction has not been investigated. Theoretically a pharmacokinetic interaction would not be anticipated.

Felbamate: The interaction has not been investigated. Theoretically a pharmacokinetic interaction could occur.

Gabapentin: Does not affect the pharmacokinetics of topiramate.

Lamotrigine: Does not affect the pharmacokinetics of topiramate.

TOPIRAMATE

Interactions with AEDs

Levetiracetam:	The interaction has not been investigated. Theoretically a pharmacokinetic interaction would not be anticipated.
	A pharmacodynamic interaction may occur whereby symptoms of decreased appetite, weight loss and nervousness present.
Oxcarbazepine:	Enhances the metabolism of topiramate.
Consequence:	Plasma topiramate levels can be decreased by 30%.
Phenobarbital:	Enhances the metabolism of topiramate.
Consequence:	Plasma topiramate levels can be decreased by up to 68%.
Phenytoin:	Enhances the metabolism of topiramate.
Consequence:	Plasma topiramate levels can be decreased by ~ 48%.
Pregabalin:	Does not affect the pharmacokinetics of topiramate.
Primidone:	Enhances the metabolism of topiramate.
Consequence:	Plasma topiramate levels can be decreased by up to 68%.
Tiagabine:	The interaction has not been investigated. Theoretically a pharmacokinetic interaction could occur.
Valproic acid:	Enhances the metabolism of topiramate.
Consequence:	Plasma topiramate levels can be decreased by up to 17%. Although this is unlikely to be of clinical significance in the majority of patients, it is noteworthy that the fraction of the hepatotoxic metabolite of valproic acid, 4-ene valproic acid, is increased.
Vigabatrin:	The interaction has not been investigated. Theoretically a pharmacokinetic interaction would not be anticipated.
Zonisamide:	The interaction has not been investigated. Theoretically a pharmacokinetic interaction would not be anticipated.

Drug Interactions Between AEDs

VALPROIC ACID

Metabolic profile

Biotransformation

The metabolism of valproic acid is both extensive and complex in that in involves multiple metabolic pathways, including ß and ω-oxidation, CYP2A6, CYP2C9, CYP2C19 and CYP2B6 isoenzymes and O-glucuronidation by UGT1A3 and UGT2B7 isoforms. To date, in excess of 25 metabolites of valproic acid have been identified. Valproic acid is an enzyme-inhibitor.

Renal excretion

Only 1-3% of a valproic acid dose is excreted in urine as unchanged valproic acid.

Pharmacokinetic characteristics

Elimination half-life of valproic acid = **7-20 hours**

New steady-state valproic acid blood levels after inhibition of valproic acid metabolism will occur **2-5 days later**.

Plasma protein binding = **90%**

Therapeutic drug monitoring

Plasma target (therapeutic) level (concentration) for valproic acid: **up to 170 μmol/L (100 μg/mL)**

Interactions with AEDs

Carbamazepine: Enhances the metabolism of valproic acid.
Consequence: Mean plasma valproic acid levels can be decreased by 39%. Co-administration with carbamazepine and other enzyme inducing AEDs does not only increase the clearance of valproic acid but may also change metabolic pathways. That patients treated with polytherapy have a greater incidence of valproic acid hepatotoxicity may be due to an increase in the 4-en and 2-4-en hepatotoxic metabolites.

Clobazam: Inhibits the metabolism of valproic acid.
Consequence: In children receiving valproic acid, clobazam decreases the clearance of valproic acid so that plasma valproic acid levels are increased.

Interactions with AEDs

Ethosuximide: Plasma valproic acid levels are decreased.

Consequence: Mean plasma valproic acid levels can be decreased by 28%. The mechanism of this interaction is unknown.

During combination therapy, ethosuximide synergistically enhances the antiepileptic efficacy (absence seizures) and toxicity of valproic acid. These effects are probably the consequence of a pharmacodynamic interaction.

Felbamate: Inhibits the metabolism of valproic acid.

Consequence: Plasma valproic acid levels can be increased by 30-50%. The interaction is the consequence of inhibition of valproic acid metabolism through ß-oxidation.

Gabapentin: Does not affect the pharmacokinetics of valproic acid.

Lamotrigine: Enhance the metabolism of valproic acid.

Consequence: Plasma valproic acid levels can be decreased by 25%.

Concurrent valproic acid therapy is a risk factor for the development of skin rash with lamotrigine. The introduction of lamotrigine to patients already taking valproic acid should be undertaken with caution, using a low starting dose and a slow does escalation rate. However, there is no risk of rash if valproic acid is introduced to patients already stabilised on lamotrigine.

During combination therapy, valproic acid synergistically enhances the antiepileptic efficacy (partial and generalised seizures) and toxicity of lamotrigine. This is considered to be the consequence of a pharmacodynamic interaction.

Levetiracetam: Does not affect the pharmacokinetics of valproic acid.

Oxcarbazepine: Does not affect the pharmacokinetics of valproic acid.

Phenobarbital: Enhances the metabolism of valproic acid.

Consequence: Co-administration with phenobarbital and other enzyme inducing AEDs does not only increase the clearance of valproic acid (mean plasma levels can be decreased by 45%) but may also change metabolic pathways. That patients treated with polytherapy have a greater incidence of valproic acid hepatotoxicity may be due to an increase in the 4-en and 2-4-en hepatotoxic metabolites.

Interactions with AEDs

Phenytoin: Enhances the metabolism of valproic acid.

Consequence: Co-administration with phenytoin and other enzyme inducing AEDs does not only increase the clearance of valproic acid (mean plasma levels are reduced by 59%) but may also change metabolic pathways. That patients treated with polytherapy have a greater incidence of valproic acid hepatotoxicity may be due to an increase in the 4-en and 2-4-en hepatotoxic metabolites.

Pregabalin: Does not affect the pharmacokinetics of valproic acid.

Primidone: Enhances the metabolism of valproic acid.

Consequence: Co-administration with primidone and other enzyme inducing AEDs does not only increase the clearance of valproic acid (mean plasma levels are reduced by 50%) but may also change metabolic pathways. That patients treated with polytherapy have a greater incidence of valproic acid hepatotoxicity may be due to an increase in the 4-en and 2-4-en hepatotoxic metabolites.

Tiagabine: Plasma valproic acid levels are decreased.

Consequence: Mean plasma levels are decreased by 10% via an unknown mechanism.

Topiramate: Enhances the metabolism of valproic acid.

Consequence: Mean plasma valproic acid levels can be decreased by 12%. This is a consequence of the induction of ß-oxidation (42%) and ω-oxidation (36%), and inhibition of the glucuronide conjugation pathway (35%). The changes in metabolite production are noteworthy, particularly since the 4-ene metabolite has been implicated as a potential hepatotoxin.

Vigabatrin: Does not affect the pharmacokinetics of valproic acid.

Zonisamide: Does not affect the pharmacokinetics of valproic acid.

VIGABATRIN

Metabolic profile

Biotransformation

Vigabatrin is not metabolised.

Renal excretion

Vigabatrin is exclusively eliminated as unchanged vigabatrin in urine.

Pharmacokinetic characteristics

Elimination half-life of vigabatrin = **5-8 hours**

New steady-state vigabatrin blood levels after inhibition of vigabatrin elimination will occur **1-2 days later.**

Plasma protein binding = **0%**

Therapeutic drug monitoring

Plasma target (therapeutic) level (concentration) for vigabatrin: **up to 280 μmol/L (36 μg/mL)**

Interactions with AEDs

Carbamazepine: Does not affect the pharmacokinetics of vigabatrin.

Ethosuximide: The interaction has not been investigated. Theoretically a pharmacokinetic interaction would not be anticipated.

Felbamate: Does not affect the pharmacokinetics of vigabatrin.

Gabapentin: The interaction has not been investigated. Theoretically a pharmacokinetic interaction would not be anticipated.

Lamotrigine: The interaction has not been investigated. Theoretically a pharmacokinetic interaction would not be anticipated.

Levetiracetam: The interaction has not been investigated. Theoretically a pharmacokinetic interaction would not be anticipated.

Oxcarbazepine: The interaction has not been investigated. Theoretically a pharmacokinetic interaction would not be anticipated.

Interactions with AEDs

Phenobarbital: Does not affect the pharmacokinetics of vigabatrin.

During combination therapy for the treatment of infantile spasms, especially in patients with tuberous sclerosis, phenobarbital appears to delay or prevent the onset of seizure control. This is considered to be the consequence of a pharmacodynamic interaction.

Phenytoin: Does not affect the pharmacokinetics of vigabatrin.

Pregabalin: The interaction has not been investigated. Theoretically a pharmacokinetic interaction would not be anticipated.

Primidone: Does not affect the pharmacokinetics of vigabatrin.

Tiagabine: The interaction has not been investigated. Theoretically a pharmacokinetic interaction would not be anticipated.

Topiramate: The interaction has not been investigated. Theoretically a pharmacokinetic interaction would not be anticipated.

Valproic acid: Does not affect the pharmacokinetics of vigabatrin.

Zonisamide: The interaction has not been investigated. Theoretically a pharmacokinetic interaction would not be anticipated.

ZONISAMIDE

Metabolic profile

Biotransformation

Zonisamide undergoes extensive metabolism, via CYP3A4, to 2-sulfamoylacetyl-phenol and subsequently to a glucuronide conjugate (50%). Also, an N-acetyl zonisamide metabolite (20%), consequent to acetylation, is formed. CYP2C19 and CYP3A5 may also contribute to the metabolism of zonisamide.

Renal excretion

Approximately 30% of zonisamide is excreted in urine as unchanged zonisamide.

Pharmacokinetic characteristics

Elimination half-life of zonisamide = **50-70 hours**

New steady-state zonisamide blood levels after inhibition of zonisamide metabolism will occur **9-18 days later.**

Plasma protein binding = **50%**

(It should be noted that felbamate also binds to erythrocytes, which have a higher affinity than plasma albumin for binding zonisamide. There is a dynamic equilibrium between free non-protein bound zonisamide and zonisamide bound to red blood cells).

Therapeutic drug monitoring

Plasma target (therapeutic) level (concentration) for zonisamide: **up to 190 μmol/L (40 μg/mL)**

Interactions with AEDs

Carbamazepine: Enhances the metabolism of zonisamide.

Consequence: Zonisamide half-life values can be decreased to ~39 hours compared to 60 hours observed in untreated volunteers. The interaction is the consequence of induction of zonisamide metabolism through CYP3A4.

Ethosuximide: The interaction has not been investigated. Theoretically a pharmacokinetic interaction would not be anticipated.

Interactions with AEDs

Felbamate:	The interaction has not been investigated. Theoretically a pharmacokinetic interaction could occur.
Gabapentin:	The interaction has not been investigated. Theoretically a pharmacokinetic interaction would not be anticipated.
Lamotrigine:	Does not affect the pharmacokinetics of zonisamide.
Levetiracetam:	The interaction has not been investigated. Theoretically a pharmacokinetic interaction would not be anticipated.
Oxcarbazepine:	The interaction has not been investigated. Theoretically a pharmacokinetic interaction could occur.
Phenobarbital:	Enhances the metabolism of zonisamide.
Consequence:	Zonisamide half-life values can be decreased to ~38 hours compared to 60 hours observed in untreated volunteers. The interaction is the consequence of induction of zonisamide metabolism through CYP3A4.
Phenytoin:	Enhances the metabolism of zonisamide.
Consequence:	Zonisamide half-life values can be decreased to ~27 hours compared to 60 hours observed in untreated volunteers. The interaction is the consequence of induction of zonisamide metabolism through CYP3A4.
Pregabalin:	The interaction has not been investigated. Theoretically a pharmacokinetic interaction would not be anticipated.
Primidone:	The interaction has not been investigated. Theoretically a pharmacokinetic interaction could occur.
Consequence:	As primidone is metabolised to phenobarbital, the same interaction as that described for phenobarbital can be expected.
Tiagabine:	The interaction has not been investigated. Theoretically a pharmacokinetic interaction would not be anticipated.
Topiramate:	The interaction has not been investigated. Theoretically a pharmacokinetic interaction could occur.
Valproic acid:	Enhances the metabolism of zonisamide.
Consequence:	Zonisamide half-life values can be decreased to ~40 hours compared to 60 hours observed in untreated volunteers. The exact mechanism of interaction is not known.
Vigabatrin:	The interaction has not been investigated. Theoretically a pharmacokinetic interaction would not be anticipated.

Table 4: Expected changes in plasma levels (concentrations) when an antiepileptic drug (AED) is added to a pre-existing AED regimen.

PRE-EXISTING AED

		CBZ	ETS	FBM	GBP	LTG	LEV	OXC	PB
	CBZ	AI	ETS⇓	FBM⇓	↔	LTG⇓	↔	H-OXC↓	↔
	ETS	↔	—	NA	NA	NA	NA	NA	↔
	FBM	CBZ↓ CBZ-E↑	?	—	NA	↔	NA	↔	PB⇑
	GBP	↔	NA	FBM↑	—	NA	↔	NA	↔
A	**LTG**	↔	↔	NA	NA	—	↔	NA	↔
E	**LEV**	↔	NA	NA	↔	↔	—	NA	↔
D	**OXC**	CBZ↓	?	?	NA	LTG↓	NA	—	PB↑
A	**PB**	CBZ⇓	ETS⇓	FBM⇓	↔	LTG⇓	↔	H-OXC↓	AI
D	**PHT**	CBZ⇓	ETS⇓	FBM⇓	↔	LTG⇓	↔	H-OXC↓	PB↑
D	**PGB**	↔	NA	NA	?	↔	↔	NA	↔
E	**PRM**	CBZ⇓	ETS⇓	FBM⇓	↔	LTG⇓	↔	?	NCC
D	**TGB**	↔	NA	NA	NA	NA	NA	NA	↔
	TPM	↔	NA	?	NA	↔	NA	?	↔
	VPA	CBZ-E⇑	ETS↑↓	FBM↑	↔	LTG⇑	↔	↔	PB⇑
	VGB	↔	NA	↔	NA	NA	NA	NA	↔
	ZNS	CBZ↑↓	NA	?	NA	↔	NA	?	↔

CBZ = carbamazepine; CBZ-E = carbamazepine-10,11-epoxide (active metabolite of CBZ); ETS = ethosuximide; FBM = felbamate; GBP = gabapentin; H-OXC = 10-hydroxycarbazepine (active metabolite of OXC); LEV = levetiracetam; LTG = lamotrigine; OXC = oxcarbazepine; PB = phenobarbital; PHT = phenytoin; PGB = pregabalin; PRM = primidone; TGB = tiagabine; TPM = topiramate; VPA = valproic acid; VGB = vigabatrin; ZNS = zonisamide.

PRE-EXISTING AED

PHT	PGB	PRM	TGB	TPM	VPA	VGB	ZNS	
PHT↑↓	↔	PRM↓ PB↑	TGB⇓	TPM⇓	VPA⇓	↔	ZNS⇓	**CBZ**
↔	NA	NA	NA	NA	VPA↓	NA	NA	**ETS**
PHT⇑	NA	?	?	?	VPA⇑	↔	?	**FBM**
↔	?	NA	NA	↔	↔	NA	NA	**GBP**
↔	↔	↔	NA	↔	↔	NA	↔	**LTG**
↔	↔	↔	NA	NA	↔	NA	NA	**LEV**
PHT↑	NA	?	?	TPM↓	↔	NA	?	**OXC**
PHT↑↓	↔	NCCP	TGB⇓	TPM⇓	VPA⇓	↔	ZNS⇓	**PB**
AI	↔	PRM↓ PB↑	TGB⇓	TPM⇓	VPA⇓	↔	ZNS⇓	**PHT**
↔	—	NA	↔	↔	↔	NA	NA	**PGB**
PHT↑↓	NA	—	TGB⇓	TPM⇓	VPA⇓	↔	ZNS⇓	**PRM**
↔	↔	↔	—	NA	↔	NA	NA	**TGB**
PHT↑	↔	↔	?	—	VPA↓	NA	?	**TPM**
PHT↓*	↔	PB⇑	↔	TPM↓	—	↔	ZNS⇓	**VPA**
PHT↓	NA	↔	NA	NA	↔	—	NA	**VGB**
PHT↑	NA	↔	NA	NA	↔	NA	—	**ZNS**

AI = autoinduction; NA = none anticipated; * free (pharmacologically active) level may increase; NCCP = not commonly co-prescribed; ↔ = No change; ↓ = a usually minor (or inconsistent) decrease in plasma level. ⇓ = a usually clinically significant decrease in plasma level; ↑ = a usually minor (or inconsistent) increase in plasma level; ⇑ = a usually clinically significant increase in plasma level. ? = The interaction has not been investigated. Theoretically a plasma level change could occur.

Drug Interactions Between AEDs and Non-AED Drugs:

CARBAMAZEPINE

Analgesics

Acetylsalicylic acid: Acetylsalicylic acid does not affect the pharmacokinetics of carbamazepine.

Dextropropoxyphene (propoxyphene): Dextropropoxyphene inhibits the metabolism of carbamazepine, probably via an action on CYP3A4. Typically plasma carbamazepine levels can increase by 40-80% but occasionally larger increases can occur (220%). Concurrent mean carbamazepine-10,11-epoxide levels can decrease by 42%.

Paracetamol: Paracetamol does not affect the pharmacokinetics of carbamazepine.

Phenylbutazone: Phenylbutazone does not affect the pharmacokinetics of carbamazepine.

Antimicrobials

Antifungal agents

Amphotericin B: Amphotericin B is not expected to affect the pharmacokinetics of carbamazepine.

Fluconazole: Fluconazole inhibits the metabolism of carbamazepine and can increase plasma carbamazepine levels. The mechanism is considered to be via an action on CYP3A4.

Flucytosine: Flucytosine is not expected to affect the pharmacokinetics of carbamazepine.

Itraconazole: The effect of itraconazole on the pharmacokinetics of carbamazepine is not known. However, itraconazole is known to inhibit CYP3A4 and therefore it may inhibit carbamazepine metabolism.

Ketoconazole: Ketoconazole inhibits the metabolism of carbamazepine and can increase plasma carbamazepine levels by 29%. Plasma carbamazepine-10,11-epoxide levels are not affected. The mechanism is considered to be via an action on CYP3A4.

Miconazole: Miconazole inhibits the metabolism of carbamazepine and can increase plasma carbamazepine levels.

Antituberculous agents

Isoniazid: Isoniazid inhibits the metabolism of carbamazepine and can result in a 45% decrease in clearance and an increase in plasma carbamazepine levels of up to 85%.

Rifampicin: Rifampicin enhances the metabolism of carbamazepine and can decrease plasma carbamazepine levels.

Antiviral agents

Delavirdine: Delavirdine inhibits the metabolism of carbamazepine, via an action on CYP3A4, and can increase plasma carbamazepine levels.

Efavirenz: Efavirenz enhances the metabolism of carbamazepine, via an action on CYP3A4, and can decrease plasma carbamazepine levels.

Indinavir: Indinavir inhibits the metabolism of carbamazepine, via an action on CYP3A4, and can increase plasma carbamazepine levels.

Nevirapine: Nevirapine enhances the metabolism of carbamazepine, via an action on CYP3A4, and can decrease plasma carbamazepine levels.

Ritonavir: Ritonavir inhibits the metabolism of carbamazepine, via an action on CYP3A4, and can increase plasma carbamazepine levels 2-3-fold.

Macrolides

Azithromycin: Azithromycin does not affect the pharmacokinetics of carbamazepine.

Clarithromycin: Clarithromycin inhibits the metabolism of carbamazepine, probably via an action on CYP3A4, and can increase plasma carbamazepine levels 2-4-fold. A concurrent decrease in plasma carbamazepine-10,11-epoxide levels can also occur.

Erythromycin: Erythromycin inhibits the metabolism of carbamazepine, probably via an action on CYP3A4, and can increase plasma carbamazepine levels 2-4-fold. Plasma carbamazepine-10,11-epoxide levels can be concurrently decreased by 40%-60%.

Drug Interactions Between AEDs and Non-AED Drugs:

Josamycin:	Josamycin inhibits the metabolism of carbamazepine, probably via an action on CYP3A4, and can increase plasma carbamazepine levels 2-4-fold.
Spiramycin:	Spiramycin does not affect the pharmacokinetics of carbamazepine.
Troleandomycin:	Troleandomycin inhibits the metabolism of carbamazepine, probably via an action on CYP3A4, and can increase plasma carbamazepine levels 2-4-fold.

Metronidazole

Metronidazole:	Metronidazole can increase plasma carbamazepine level by ~ 60%. The mechanism of this interaction is not known.

Antineoplastic agents

Cisplatin:	Cisplatin may decrease plasma carbamazepine levels.

Antiulcer drugs

Antacids and surface acting drugs

Antacids:	Antacids can reduce the absorption of carbamazepine resulting in decreased plasma carbamazepine levels. This interaction can be avoided by separating the administration of carbamazepine and antacids by at least 2 hours.

Histamine H_2–receptor antagonists

Cimetidine:	Cimetidine inhibits the metabolism of carbamazepine, via an action on CYP3A4, and can increase carbamazepine half-life values by 18%, AUC values by 26% and plasma carbamazepine levels can be increased by ~30%. In many patients this interaction is transient.
Famotidine:	Famotidine does not affect the pharmacokinetics of carbamazepine.
Ranitidine:	Ranitidine does not affect the pharmacokinetics of carbamazepine.

Proton pump inhibitors

Omeprazole: Conflicting effects have been reported. A multiple-dose study of healthy volunteers found a 42% increase in plasma carbamazepine levels during concurrent omeprazole administration. However, a patient study has reported that omeprazole was without effect on plasma carbamazepine levels. It should be noted that the contribution of CYP3A4 to the metabolism of omeprazole is minimal and also there is evidence to suggest that it neither induces nor inhibits CYP3A4 activity.

Pantoprazole: Pantoprazole does not affect the pharmacokinetics of carbamazepine.

Cardiovascular drugs

Antiarrhythmics

Amiodarone: Amiodarone does not affect the pharmacokinetics of carbamazepine.

Antihypertensive agents

Diltiazem: Diltiazem inhibits the metabolism of carbamazepine and can increase plasma carbamazepine levels by 56%.

Nifedipine: Nifedipine does not affect the pharmacokinetics of carbamazepine.

Nimodipine: Nimodipine does not affect the pharmacokinetics of carbamazepine.

Verapamil: Verapamil inhibits the metabolism of carbamazepine and can increase plasma carbamazepine levels by 40%-60%. Plasma carbamazepine-10,11-epoxide levels are unaffected.

Antiplatelet drugs

Ticlopidine: Ticlopidine inhibits the metabolism of carbamazepine, perhaps via an action on CYP3A4, and can increase plasma carbamazepine levels by up to 74%.

Drug Interactions Between AEDs and Non-AED Drugs:

CARBAMAZEPINE

Lipid lowering drugs

Colestipol: Colestipol can reduce the absorption of carbamazepine by 10%.

Colestyramine: Colestyramine does not affect the pharmacokinetics of carbamazepine.

Gemfibrozil: Plasma carbamazepine levels can be increased by 30-65%. The suggested mechanism is that the clearance of carbamazepine is increased in those patients with elevated cholesterol and total lipids, thus when the condition is treated with gemfibrozil, clearance becomes more normal resulting in an increase in plasma carbamazepine levels.

Oral anticoagulants

Pentoxifylline: Pentoxifylline does not affect the pharmacokinetics of carbamazepine.

Herbal remedies

Anthranoid-containing plants

Plants such as senna (Cassia senna) and cascara (Rhamnus purshiana), and soluble fibres (including Guar gum and Psyllium) are known to decrease the absorption of a variety of drugs and potential interactions between these products and carbamazepine (and indeed other AEDs) needs to be considered.

St John's Wort (Hypericum perforatum)

St John's Wort can enhance the metabolism of carbamazepine, by inducing CYP3A4 and possibly also by affecting the activity of drug trasporters in the gastrointestinal tract. Indeed, St John's Wort has been shown to decrease plasma carbamazepine levels after a single-dose of carbamazepine, although no interaction was identified at steady-state.

Immunosuppressants

Cyclosporine A: Cyclosporine A does not affect the pharmacokinetics of carbamazepine.

Sirolimus: Sirolimus does not affect the pharmacokinetics of carbamazepine.

Tacrolimus: Tacrolimus does not affect the pharmacokinetics of carbamazepine.

Psychotropic drugs

Antidepressants

Citalopram: Citalopram does not affect the pharmacokinetics of carbamazepine.

Fluoxetine: Fluoxetine can increase plasma carbamazepine levels. However, the interaction appears to be variable with plasma levels of carbamazepine and its metabolite, carbamazepine-10,11-epoxide, ranging from no effect to a 30% increase in levels.

Fluvoxamine: Fluvoxamine can increase plasma carbamazepine levels. However, the interaction appears to be variable with plasma levels of carbamazepine and its metabolite, carbamazepine-10, 11-epoxide, ranging from no effect to a 70% increase in levels.

Nefazodone: Nefazodone can increase plasma carbamazepine levels by up to 3-fold. A concurrent decrease in plasma carbamazepine-10,11-epoxide levels is also observed.

Paroxetine: Paroxetine does not affect the pharmacokinetics of carbamazepine.

Sertraline: Sertraline does not affect the pharmacokinetics of carbamazepine.

Trazodone: Trazodone can increase plasma carbamazepine levels by 26%.

Viloxazine: Viloxazine can increase plasma carbamazepine levels by 55% and plasma carbamazepine-10,11-epoxide levels by 16%.

Antipsychotics

Haloperidol: Haloperidol can increase plasma carbamazepine levels by 42%.

Loxapine: Loxapine does not affect plasma carbamazepine levels. However, plasma carbamazepine-10,11-epoxide levels can be increased.

Quetiapine: Quetiapine does not affect plasma carbamazepine levels. However, plasma carbamazepine-10,11-epoxide levels can be increased 3-4-fold.

Risperidone: Risperidone can increase plasma carbamazepine levels, probably via inhibition of CYP3A4, by 10%.

Thioridazine: Thioridazine does not affect the pharmacokinetics of carbamazepine.

Steroids

Danazol: Danazol inhibits the metabolism of carbamazepine and can increase plasma carbamazepine levels by 50-100%.

Miscellanea

Disulfiram: Disulfiram does not affect the pharmacokinetics of carbamazepine.

CLOBAZAM

Cimetidine: Cimetidine can increase plasma clobazam levels by ~ 17%. In contrast, plasma N-desmethylclobazam levels (the pharmacologically active metabolite of clobazam) are unaffected.

Drug Interactions Between AEDs and Non-AED Drugs:

CLONAZEPAM

Amiodarone:	Clonazepam toxicity was observed in a patient co-prescribed amiodarone, which resolved upon clonazepam withdrawal. The mechanism of this interaction is unknown.
Fluoxetine:	Fluoxetine does not affect the pharmacokinetics of clonazepam.
Ritonavir:	Ritonavir inhibits the metabolism of clonazepam, via an action on CYP3A4, and can increase plasma carbamazepine levels 3-fold.
Sertraline:	Sertraline does not affect the pharmacokinetics of clonazepam.

ETHOSUXIMIDE

Antimicrobials
Antituberculous agents

Isoniazid: Isoniazid inhibits the metabolism of ethosuximide and can increase plasma ethosuximide levels 4-fold.

Rifampicin: Rifampicin enhances the metabolism of ethosuximide and can decrease plasma ethosuximide levels.

Antiviral agents

Ritonavir: Ritonavir inhibits the metabolism of ethosuximide, via an action on CYP3A4, and can increase plasma ethosuximide levels.

FELBAMATE

Antimicrobials
Macrolides
Erythromycin: Erythromycin does not affect the pharmacokinetics of felbamate.

Antiulcer drugs
Antacids and surface acting drugs
Antacids: Concurrent administration of antacids (Maalox Plus; aluminium/magnesium hydroxides) does not affect the rate or extent of felbamate absorption.

GABAPENTIN

Antacids: Antacids (Maalox; aluminium hydroxide/magnesium hydroxide) can reduce the oral bioavailability of gabapentin by 20%. To avoid problems, administration of gabapentin and antacids should be separated by at least 2 hours.

Cimetidine: Cimetidine can decrease the oral clearance of gabapentin by 14%.

Probenecid: Probenecid does not affect the pharmacokinetics of gabapentin.

LAMOTRIGINE

Analgesics

Acetaminophen: Acetaminophen can decrease plasma lamotrigine AUC values by 20% and elimination half-life values by 15% and enhances the urinary elimination of lamotrigine via an unknown mechanism.

Antimicrobials

Antituberculous agents

Rifampicin: Rifampicin enhances the metabolism of lamotrigine, via an action on glucuronidation, and can decrease plasma lamotrigine AUC values by 44%.

Antiviral agents

Ritonavir: Ritonavir can enhance the metabolism of lamotrigine, via induction of UDP-glucuronyltransferases, and can decrease plasma lamotrigine levels.

Zidovudine: Because zidovudine undergoes metabolism via glucuronidation, it is theoretically possible that zidovudine may affect the pharmacokinetics of lamotrigine.

Antiulcer drugs

Histamine H2-receptor antagonists

Cimetidine: Cimetidine does not affect the pharmacokinetics of lamotrigine.

Psychotropic drugs

Antidepressants

Sertraline: Sertraline can increase plasma lamotrigine levels 2-fold. Inhibition of lamotrigine glucuronidation by sertraline has been proposed to explain this interaction.

Paroxetine: Paroxetine does not affect the pharmacokinetics of lamotrigine.

Steroids

Oral contraceptives: Oral contraceptives enhance the metabolism of lamotrigine and can decrease plasma lamotrigine levels by 40-65%.

Miscellanea

Bupropion: Bupropion does not affect the pharmacokinetics of lamotrigine.

LEVETIRACETAM

Digoxin: Digoxin does not affect the pharmacokinetics of levetiracetam.

Probenecid: Probenecid does not affect the pharmacokinetics of levetiracetam. However, the plasma level of its primary non-pharmacologically active metabolite, ucbLO59, increases 2.5-fold consequent to a 61% decrease in tubular excretion.

Warfarin: Warfarin does not affect the pharmacokinetics of levetiracetam.

OXCARBAZEPINE

Analgesics

Dextropropoxyphene (propoxyphene): Dextropropoxyphene does not affect the pharmacokinetics of oxcarbazepine.

Antimicrobials

Macrolides

Erythromycin: Erythromycin does not affect the pharmacokinetics of oxcarbazepine.

Antiulcer drugs

Histamine H$_2$-receptor antagonists

Cimetidine: Cimetidine does not affect the pharmacokinetics of oxcarbazepine.

Cardioactive drugs

Antihypertensive agents

Verapamil: Verapamil can decrease plasma 10-hydroxycarbazepine (the pharmacologically active metabolite of oxcarbazepine) levels by 20%.

Psychotropic drugs

Antidepressant

Viloxazine: Viloxazine can increase plasma 10-hydroxycarbazepine levels by 15%.

PHENOBARBITAL

Analgesics

Dextropropoxyphene (propoxyphene): Dextropropoxyphene can increase plasma phenobarbital levels by 20%.

Antimicrobials

Chloramphenicol: Chloramphenicol inhibits the metabolism of phenobarbital and can increase plasma phenobarbital levels.

Antiulcer drugs

Antacids and surface acting drugs

Antacids: Phenobarbital absorption is significantly reduced by concurrent administration of antacids. To avoid problems, administration of phenobarbital and antacids should be separated by at least 2 hours.

Histamine H_2–receptor antagonists

Cimetidine: Cimetidine does not affect the pharmacokinetics of phenobarbital.

Cardioactive drugs

Oral anticoagulants

Dicoumarol: Dicoumarol can increase plasma phenobarbital levels.

Miscellanea

Disulfiram: Disulfiram does not affect the pharmacokinetics of phenobarbital.

Drug Interactions Between AEDs and Non-AED Drugs:

PHENYTOIN

Analgesics

Aspirin: Salicylates displace phenytoin from its plasma protein binding sites (primarily albumin). A 27% increase in the phenytoin free fraction and a 20% decrease in total phenytoin AUC values can be expected but free (non-protein bound) phenytoin AUC values are unchanged. Although no change in clinical effect of phenytoin is expected, a change in the interpretation of total plasma phenytoin level measurements may be required. In this setting clinical management may best be guided by measurement of free phenytoin levels.

Dextropropoxyphene (propoxyphene): Dextropropoxyphene can increase plasma phenytoin levels. This interaction is consistent with in vitro and clinical reports of inhibition of other CYP2C9 substrates by dextropropoxyphene.

Fenyramidol: Fenyramidol inhibits the metabolism of phenytoin and can increase plasma phenytoin levels by 40-200%.

Ibuprofen: Ibuprofen does not affect the pharmacokinetics of phenytoin.

Paracetamol: Paracetamol does not affect the pharmacokinetics of phenytoin.

Phenylbutazone: The interaction between phenylbutazone and phenytoin is complex in that initially plasma phenytoin levels can decrease (~20%) and then they increase. The mechanism of this interaction involves a concurrent plasma protein binding displacement interaction and an inhibition of phenytoin metabolism by phenylbutazone.

Antimicrobials

Atovaquone

Atovaquone: Atovaquone does not affect the pharmacokinetics of phenytoin.

Antifungal agents

Amphotericin B: Amphotericin B does not affect the pharmacokinetics of phenytoin.

Fluconazole: Fluconazole can increase plasma phenytoin levels by 2-4-fold.

Flucytosine:	Flucytosine is not expected to affect the pharmacokinetics of phenytoin.
Itraconazole:	Itraconazole can increase plasma phenytoin levels by ~ 10%.
Ketoconazole:	Ketoconazole does not affect the pharmacokinetics of phenytoin.
Miconazole:	Miconazole can increase plasma phenytoin levels by 2-4-fold.
Voriconazole:	Voriconazole inhibits the metabolism of phenytoin, via an action on CYP2C9, and can increase phenytoin AUC values by 80% and plasma phenytoin levels by 70%.

Antituberculous agents

Isoniazid:	Isoniazid can inhibit the metabolism of phenytoin resulting in a 3-fold increase in plasma phenytoin levels. However, this interaction is only relevant in those patients that are "slow metabolizers (acetylators)" of isoniazid (which is genetically determined) and attain sufficiently high plasma isoniazid levels so as to inhibit the metabolism of phenytoin.
Rifampicin:	Rifampicin enhances the metabolism of phenytoin and can increase phenytoin clearance by up to 109%.
	When rifampicin and isoniazid are administered in combination, rifampicin counteracts the inhibiting effect of isoniazid on phenytoin metabolism.

Antiviral agents

Acyclovir:	Acyclovir can decrease plasma phenytoin levels by 70%. The exact mechanism of this interaction is not known but is considered to be an effect on gastrointestinal absorption.
Indinavir:	Indinavir inhibits the metabolism of phenytoin and can increase plasma phenytoin levels.
Nelfinavir:	Nelfinavir inhibits the metabolism of phenytoin and can increase plasma phenytoin levels.
Ritonavir:	Ritonavir inhibits the metabolism of phenytoin and can increase plasma phenytoin levels.

Drug Interactions Between AEDs and Non-AED Drugs:

Saquinavir: Saquinavir inhibits the metabolism of phenytoin and can increase plasma phenytoin levels.

Zidovudine: Zidovudine does not affect the pharmacokinetics of phenytoin.

Chloramphenicol

Chloramphenicol: Chloramphenicol inhibits the metabolism of phenytoin and can increase phenytoin elimination half-life values and plasma phenytoin levels 1-3-fold.

Fluoroquinolones

Clinafloxacin: Clinafloxacin can increase plasma phenytoin levels by 15%.

Ciprofloxacin: There have been conflicting data on a possible interaction of ciprofloxacin with phenytoin, with no change, a decrease or an increase in plasma phenytoin levels having all been reported.

Isotretinoin

Isotretinoin: Isotretinoin does not affect the pharmacokinetics of phenytoin.

Macrolides

Clarithromycin: Clarithromycin can increase plasma phenytoin levels by 2-fold.

Erythromycin: There have been conflicting data on a possible interaction of erythromycin with phenytoin, with no change or an increase in plasma phenytoin levels having been reported.

Metronidazole

Metronidazole: Metronidazole inhibits the metabolism of phenytoin and can decrease phenytoin clearance by 15% and increases plasma phenytoin levels.

Sulfonamides

Cotrimoxazole: Cotrimoxazole (a mixture of sulfamethoxazole and trimethoprim) inhibits the metabolism of phenytoin and can increase plasma phenytoin levels.

Sulfaphenazole: Sulfaphenazole and to a lesser extent other sulfonamides (e.g. sulfadiazine, sulfamethizole, salfamethoxazole), may inhibit phenytoin metabolism and increase plasma phenytoin levels. Some of these sulfonamides concurrently displace phenytoin from plasma protein binding sites (primarily albumin), and therefore measurement of total phenytoin level may underestimate the increase in the level of the free, pharmacologically active drug. In this setting, patient management may benefit from monitoring free phenytoin levels.

Sulfadimethoxine: Sulfadimethoxine does not affect the pharmacokinetics of phenytoin.

Sulfmethoxudiazine: Sulfmethoxudiazine does not affect the pharmacokinetics of phenytoin.

Sulfamethoxy-pyridazine: Sulfamethoxypyridazine does not affect the pharmacokinetics of phenytoin.

Antineoplastic agents

Bleomycin: Bleomycin can significantly decrease plasma phenytoin levels but this may be a consequence of antineoplastic damage to the intestinal mucosa and impaired phenytoin absorption. Only 22% of a phenytoin dose is absorbed during combination therapy with cisplatin, vinblastine and bleomycin.

Carboplatin: Carboplatin can decrease plasma phenytoin levels by 50%. This interaction may be the consequence of enhanced hepatic metabolism or a displacement of phenytoin from its plasma protein binding sites.

Carmustine: Carmustine can decrease plasma phenytoin levels by 50%.

Cisplatin: Cisplatin can decrease plasma phenytoin levels by more than 50%. Cisplatin possibly enhances the metabolism of phenytoin although a change in volume of distribution could also be responsible for this interaction. During combination treatment with cisplatin, vinblastine and bleomycin plasma phenytoin levels can be decreased as a result of a 78% reduction of phenytoin absorption. Damage to the intestinal mucosa is probably the mechanism of this interaction.

Doxifluridine: Doxifluridine inhibits the metabolism of phenytoin and can increase plasma phenytoin levels 4-fold.

Drug Interactions Between AEDs and Non-AED Drugs:

Etoposide: Etoposide enhances the metabolism of phenytoin and can decrease plasma phenytoin levels.

5-Fluorouracil: 5-Fluorouracil inhibits the metabolism of phenytoin, via an action on CYP3A9, and can increase plasma phenytoin levels.

Methotrexate: Methotrexate can decrease plasma phenytoin levels but this may be a consequence of antineoplastic damage to the intestinal mucosa and impaired phenytoin absorption.

Tegafur: Tegafur inhibits the metabolism of phenytoin and can increase plasma phenytoin levels.

Tamoxifen: Tamoxifen can increase plasma phenytoin levels by 44%. The mechanism of this interaction is unknown.

UFT: UFT (a mixture of uracil and the 5-fluorouracil pro-drug tegafur) inhibits the metabolism of phenytoin and can increase plasma phenytoin levels.

Vinblastine: Vinblastine can decrease plasma phenytoin levels by ~50%. This interaction may be a consequence of antineoplastic damage to the intestinal mucosa and impaired phenytoin absorption. During combination treatment with cisplatin, vinblastine and bleomycin, as little as 22% of a phenytoin dose is absorbed.

Antiulcer drugs

Antacids and surface acting drugs

Antacids: A significant reduction in phenytoin absorption can occur when phenytoin is co-ingested with calcium-containing and aluminium hydroxide-magnesium salt antacids. However, this has not been a consistent finding in all studies. Factors affecting the extent of interaction include antacid dose, administration times, motility of gastrointestinal tract, and plasma phenytoin levels. To avoid this interaction the administration of phenytoin and antacids should be separated by at least 2 hours.

Sucralfate: Phenytoin bioavailability can be reduced by 20-30% by sucralfate, but the interaction is avoided when phenytoin is ingested at least 2 hours before sucralfate ingestion.

Histamine H$_2$–receptor antagonists

Cimetidine: Cimetidine inhibits the metabolism of phenytoin, via an action on CYP2C19, and can increase plasma phenytoin levels by 37%.

Famotidine: Famotidine does not affect the pharmacokinetics of phenytoin.

Nizatidine: Nizatidine does not affect the pharmacokinetics of phenytoin.

Ranitidine: With the exception of an isolated case report where phenytoin plasma levels were increased by 50%, ranitidine has not been found to affect the pharmacokinetics of phenytoin.

Proton pump inhibitors

Esomeprazole: Esomeprazole inhibits the metabolism of phenytoin, via an action on CYP2C19, and can increase plasma phenytoin levels by < 25%.

Lansoprazole: Lansoprazole does not affect the pharmacokinetics of phenytoin.

Omeprazole: Omeprazole inhibits the metabolism of phenytoin, via an action on CYP2C19, and can increase plasma phenytoin levels by 25%.

Pantoprazole: Pantoprazole does not affect the pharmacokinetics of phenytoin.

Rabeprazole: Rabeprazole does not affect the pharmacokinetics of phenytoin.

Cardiovascular drugs

Antiarrhythmics

Amiodarone: Amiodarone inhibits the metabolism of phenytoin and can increase plasma phenytoin levels 3-4-fold.

Antihypertensive agents

Diazoxide: Diazoxide enhances the metabolism of phenytoin and can decrease plasma phenytoin levels.

Diltiazem: Diltiazem can increase plasma phenytoin levels by 90%.

Losartan: Losartan does not affect the pharmacokinetics of phenytoin.

Nifedipine: Nifedipine can increase plasma phenytoin levels.

Verapamil: Verapamil can increase plasma phenytoin levels.

Drug Interactions Between AEDs and Non-AED Drugs:

Antiplatelet drugs

Ticlopidine: Ticlopidine inhibits the metabolism of phenytoin, via an action on CYP2C19, and can increase plasma phenytoin levels 4.5-fold.

Digoxin

Digoxin: Digoxin does not affect the pharmacokinetics of phenytoin.

Lipid lowering drugs

Colestipol: Colestipol does not affect the pharmacokinetics of phenytoin.

Colestyramine: Colestyramine does not affect the pharmacokinetics of phenytoin.

Oral anticoagulants

Dicoumarol: Dicoumarol can increase plasma phenytoin levels.

Warfarin: Warfarin does not affect the pharmacokinetics of phenytoin.

Herbal remedies

Anthranoid-containing plants: Plants such as senna (Cassia senna) and cascara (Rhamnus purshiana), and soluble fibres (including Guar gum and Psyllium) are known to decrease the absorption of a variety of drugs and potential interactions between these products and phenytoin (and indeed other AEDs) needs to be considered.

Ayurvedic syrup shankhapushpi: A reduction in plasma phenytoin levels and a lowering of seizure threshold has been reported after intake of Ayurvedic syrup shankhapushpi.

Evening primrose oil: A reduction in plasma phenytoin levels and a lowering of seizure threshold has been reported after intake of Evening primrose oil.

St John's Wort (Hypericum perforatum):   St John's Wort has the potential to increase the metabolism of phenytoin, by inducing CYP2C9 and possibly also by affecting the activity of drug transporters in the gastrointestinal tract.

Psychotropic drugs

Antidepressants

Imipramine: Imipramine has been associated with an increase in plasma phenytoin levels in some reports; however, others observed no changes.

Fluoxetine: Fluoxetine inhibits the metabolism of phenytoin, via an action on CYP2C9, and can increase plasma phenytoin levels by up to 4-fold.

Fluvoxamine: Fluvoxamine can increase plasma phenytoin levels by 3-fold.

Mirtazepine: Mirtazepine does not affect the pharmacokinetics of phenytoin.

Nefazodone: The pharmacokinetics of phenytoin was not altered when given as a single dose to healthy subjects receiving nefazodone. However, further study with chronic administration and higher phenytoin doses is needed to rule out an interaction between these drugs.

Paroxetine: Paroxetine does not affect the pharmacokinetics of phenytoin.

Sertraline: Sertraline inhibits the metabolism of phenytoin, via an action on CYP2C9, and can increase plasma phenytoin levels 6-fold.

Trazodone: A patient experienced a 2.5-fold increase in plasma phenytoin levels and toxicity during concurrent administration of phenytoin and trazodone. Further evaluation of this interaction is needed.

Venlafaxine: Venlafaxine does not affect the pharmacokinetics of phenytoin.

Viloxazine: Viloxazine inhibits the metabolism of phenytoin and can increase plasma phenytoin levels by 50%.

Antipsychotics

Chlorpromazine: There have been conflicting data on a possible interaction of chlorpromazine with phenytoin, with no change, a decrease or an increase in plasma phenytoin level having all been reported.

Haloperidol: Haloperidol does not affect the pharmacokinetics of phenytoin.

Loxapine: Loxapine can decrease plasma phenytoin levels.

Drug Interactions Between AEDs and Non-AED Drugs:

Risperidone: Risperidone inhibits the metabolism phenytoin, probably via an action on CYP2C9, and can increase plasma phenytoin levels by 20%.

Thioridazine: An increase in plasma phenytoin levels and neurotoxicity was reported in 2 patients after the addition of thioridazine. However, a crossover study in 7 patients with epilepsy found no change in plasma phenytoin levels after 6 weeks of thioridazine administration.

Steroids

Dexamethasone: Dexamethasone therapy can be associated with a 50% decrease in plasma phenytoin levels. In one study an unexpected increase (mean 38%) in plasma phenytoin levels has been reported.

Danazol: Danazol does not affect the pharmacokinetics of phenytoin.

Miscellanea

Allopurinol: Allopurinol inhibits the metabolism of phenytoin and can increase AUC values by 50-120% and plasma phenytoin levels can increase by 26-37%.

Azapropazone: Azapropazone inhibits the metabolism of phenytoin and can decrease phenytoin clearance by 35-59% and can increase plasma phenytoin levels at least 2-fold.

Chlorphenamine (chlorpheniramine): Chlorphenamine inhibits phenytoin metabolism and can increase plasma phenytoin levels.

Disulfiram: Disulfiram inhibits the metabolism of phenytoin and can increase plasma phenytoin levels by up to 5-fold.

Methylphenidate: Methylphenidate inhibits the metabolism of phenytoin and can increase plasma phenytoin levels.

Orlistat: Orlistat does not affect the pharmacokinetics of phenytoin.

Phenylbutazone: Phenylbutazone inhibits the metabolism of phenytoin and can increase phenytoin elimination half-life values and plasma phenytoin levels.

Sulfinpyrazone: Sulfinpyrazone inhibits the metabolism of phenytoin and can increase plasma phenytoin levels 2-fold.

Theophylline: Theophylline can decrease phenytoin plasma levels by 21%. The interaction may be attributable to decreased oral absorption.

Tolbutamide: Tolbutamide can cause a transient 45% increase in free non-protein bound plasma phenytoin levels.

Zileuton: Zileuton does not affect the pharmacokinetics of phenytoin.

PREGABALIN

There have been no reports on the effect of non-AED drugs on the pharmacokinetics of pregabalin.

PRIMIDONE

Antimicrobials

Antituberculous agents

Isoniazid: Isoniazid inhibits the metabolism of primidone and can increase plasma primidone levels by 83% and decrease plasma phenobarbital levels by 12%. The elimination half-life of primidone can increase by 60%.

General note: As primidone is metabolised to phenobarbital, all the interactions highlighted for phenobarbital will also apply to primidone.

TIAGABINE

Antimicrobials

Macrolides

Clarithromycin: Although no clinical studies have been undertaken, the fact that clarithromycin is an inhibitor of CYP3A4 and since this isoenzyme is involved in the metabolism of tiagabine, the possibility of an increase in plasma tiagabine levels should be considered during co-administration.

Erythromycin: Erythromycin does not affect the pharmacokinetics of tiagabine.

Troleandomycin: Although no clinical studies have been undertaken, the fact that troleandomycin is an inhibitor of CYP3A4 and since this isoenzyme is involved in the metabolism of tiagabine, the possibility of an increase in plasma tiagabine levels should be considered during co-administration.

Antiulcer drugs

Histamine H_2-receptor antagonists

Cimetidine: Cimetidine does not affect the pharmacokinetics of tiagabine.

Triazolam: Triazolam does not affect the pharmacokinetics of tiagabine.

Cardiovascular drugs

Digoxin: Digoxin does not affect the pharmacokinetics of tiagabine.

Oral anticoagulants

Warfarin: Warfarin does not affect the pharmacokinetics of tiagabine.

Miscellanea

Theophylline: Theophylline does not affect the pharmacokinetics of tiagabine.

TOPIRAMATE

Cardioactive drugs

Propranolol: Propranolol can decrease topiramate clearance values by 8-14% and increase plasma topiramate levels by 9-16%.

Psychoactive drugs

Antidepressants

Amitriptyline: Amitriptyline can decrease the clearance of topiramate.

Lithium: Lithium can decrease the clearance of topiramate.

Miscellanea

Dihydroergotamine: Dihydroergotamine does not affect the pharmacokinetics of topiramate.

Sumatriptan: Sumatriptan can decrease the clearance of topiramate.

VALPROIC ACID

Analgesics

Aspirin: Salicylates displace valproic acid from plasma protein binding sites (primarily albumin) and can inhibit valproic acid metabolism, via the ß-oxidation pathway, by 66%. Concurrent administration of an antipyretic dose of aspirin to children can result in a 23% increase in free non-protein bound plasma valproic acid levels. As total plasma valproic acid levels would underestimate the level of free (pharmacologically active) valproic acid, there may be advantages in managing patients by monitoring free valproic acid levels.

Antimicrobials

Aminoglycosides

Amikacin: Amikacin can decrease plasma valproic acid levels, probably via an induction of valproic acid metabolism.

Beta-lactams

Meropenem: Meropenem can decrease plasma valproic acid levels. There is preliminary evidence to suggest that the mechanism of this interaction involves inhibition of the gastrointestinal absorption of valproic acid.

Paripenem: Paripenem can decrease plasma valproic acid levels. There is preliminary evidence to suggest that the mechanism of this interaction involves inhibition of the gastrointestinal absorption of valproic acid.

Antituberculous agents

Isoniazid: Isoniazid can inhibit the metabolism of valproic acid and increase plasma valproic acid levels.

Rifampicin: Rifampicin enhances the metabolism of valproic acid and can increase valproic acid clearance by 40% and decreases plasma valproic acid levels.

Antiviral agents

Acyclovir: Acyclovir can decrease plasma valproic acid levels by 80%. The exact mechanism of this interaction is not known but is thought to be an effect on gastrointestinal absorption.

Ritonavir: Ritonavir enhances the metabolism of valproic acid, via induction of glucuronyl transferases, and can decrease plasma valproic levels.

Macrolides

Erythromycin: A single case of an increase in valproic acid plasma levels and toxicity following the addition of erythromycin has been reported. The lack of other reports, with what is probably a relatively common drug combination, suggests that most patients tolerate the concurrent administration of these two drugs without problems.

Antineoplastic agents

Cisplatin: Cisplatin can decrease plasma valproic acid levels.

Efavirenz: Efavirenz does not affect the pharmacokinetics of valproic acid.

Lopinavir: Lopinavir does not affect the pharmacokinetics of valproic acid.

Methotrexate: Methotrexate can decrease plasma valproic acid levels by 75%. The exact mechanism is unknown; possible mechanisms include plasma protein binding displacement or a decrease in valproic acid absorption.

Antiulcer drugs

Antacids and surface acting drugs

A single-dose study in healthy volunteers evaluated the effect of three antacid preparations on valproic acid absorption. Whilst no significant change in extent of absorption occurred with some antacids (e.g. aluminium hydroxide/magnesium trisilicate, or calcium carbonate), concurrent administration of another (aluminium hydroxide/magnesium hydroxide) produced a small (12%) but statistically significant increase in valproic acid AUC values.

Drug Interactions Between AEDs and Non-AED Drugs:

Histamine H$_2$–receptor antagonists

Cimetidine:	Cimetidine does not affect the pharmacokinetics of valproic acid.
Ranitidine:	Ranitidine does not affect the pharmacokinetics of valproic acid.

Cardioactive drugs

Colestyramine:	Colestyramine can decrease the absorption of valproic acid by 15%.
Propranolol:	Propranolol does not affect the pharmacokinetics of valproic acid.

Psychoactive drugs

Antidepressants

Lithium:	Lithium can increase valproic acid AUC values by 11 % and plasma valproic acid levels by 7%. A pharmacodynamic interaction, leading to neurotoxic symptoms in patients receiving lithium in combination with valproic acid has been reported.
Fluoxetine:	Anecdotal reports in two patients suggest that fluoxetine causes an increase in valproic acid plasma levels. In contrast, two cases of decreased plasma valproic acid levels have also been reported.
Paroxetine:	Paroxetine does not affect the pharmacokinetics of valproic acid.
Sertraline:	Sertraline can increase plasma valproic acid levels.
Venlafaxine:	Venlafaxine does not affect the pharmacokinetics of valproic acid.

Antipsychotics

Chlorpromazine:	Chlorpromazine can decrease valproic acid clearance values by 14%, increase elimination half-life values by 14% and increase plasma valproic acid levels by 22%.
Haloperidol:	Haloperidol does not affect the pharmacokinetics of valproic acid.

Steroids

Danazol:	Danazol does not affect the pharmacokinetics of valproic acid.

Miscellanea

Diflunisal: Diflunisal can increase the clearance of valproic acid and decrease plasma valproic acid levels. These changes are not the consequence of a metabolic interaction (glucuronidation and/or ß-oxidation) but that of an effect at the renal level whereby diflunisal interferes with the renal excretion of at least 3 of the metabolites of valproic acid.

Naproxen: Naproxen enhances the metabolism of valproic acid, via an action on glucuronidation, and can increase valproic acid clearance by 20%.

Theophylline: Theophylline does not affect the pharmacokinetics of valproic acid.

VIGABATRIN

There have been no reports on the effects of non-AED drugs on the pharmacokinetics of vigabatrin.

ZONISAMIDE

Antimicrobials
Antiviral agents
Ritonavir: Ritonavir does not affect the pharmacokinetics of zonisamide.

Antiulcer drugs
Histamine H_2-receptor antagonists
Cimetidine: Cimetidine does not affect the pharmacokinetics of zonisamide.

Psychotropic drugs
Antipsychotics
Risperidone: Risperidone can decrease plasma zonisamide levels.

Miscellanea

In vitro studies show that zonisamide metabolism is markedly inhibited by cyclosporine A, dihydroergotamine, ketoconazole, itraconazole, miconazole and triazolam. Therefore, the possibility exists that in the clinical setting these drugs may interfere with the metabolism of zonisamide if co-prescribed.

Drug Interactions Between AEDs and Non-AED Drugs:

ANALGESICS

Fentanyl

Carbamazepine: Carbamazepine enhances the metabolism of fentanyl so that a higher fentanyl dosage is required in order to maintain anaesthesia.

Phenobarbital: Phenobarbital enhances the metabolism of fentanyl so that a higher fentanyl dosage is required in order to maintain anaesthesia.

Phenytoin: Phenytoin enhances the metabolism of fentanyl so that a higher fentanyl dosage is required in order to maintain anaesthesia.

Primidone: Primidone enhances the metabolism of fentanyl so that a higher fentanyl dosage is required in order to maintain anaesthesia.

Meperidine

Carbamazepine: Carbamazepine enhances the metabolism of meperidine so that plasma meperidine levels are decreased whilst plasma levels of normeperidine, its pharmacologically active metabolite that has a lower analgesic potency but greater toxicity than meperidine, are increased.

Phenobarbital: Phenobarbital enhances the metabolism of meperidine so that plasma meperidine levels are decreased whilst plasma levels of normeperidine, its pharmacologically active metabolite that has a lower analgesic potency but greater toxicity than meperidine, are increased.

Phenytoin: Phenytoin enhances the metabolism of meperidine so that plasma meperidine levels are decreased whilst plasma levels of normeperidine, its pharmacologically active metabolite that has a lower analgesic potency but greater toxicity than meperidine, are increased.

Primidone: Primidone enhances the metabolism of meperidine so that plasma meperidine levels are decreased whilst plasma levels of normeperidine, its pharmacologically active metabolite that has a lower analgesic potency but greater toxicity than meperidine, are increased.

Methadone

Carbamazepine: Carbamazepine enhances the metabolism of methadone and can decrease plasma methadone levels.

Phenobarbital: Phenobarbital enhances the metabolism of methadone and can decrease plasma methadone levels.

Phenytoin: Phenytoin enhances the metabolism of methadone and can decrease plasma methadone levels.

Paracetamol

Carbamazepine: Carbamazepine enhances the metabolism of paracetamol, probably via an action on CYP1A2, and can decrease paracetamol AUC values by 40% and increase its clearance by 52%.

Phenobarbital: Phenobarbital enhances the metabolism of paracetamol, probably via an action on CYP1A2, and can decrease paracetamol AUC values by 40% and increase its clearance by 52%.

Phenytoin: Phenytoin enhances the metabolism of paracetamol, probably via an action on CYP1A2, and can decrease paracetamol AUC values by 40% and increase its clearance by 52%. Plasma paracetamol levels can be decreased by up to 75%.

Primidone: Primidone enhances the metabolism of paracetamol, probably via an action on CYP1A2, and can decrease paracetamol AUC values by 40% and increase its clearance by 52%.

Pethidine

Phenytoin: Phenytoin enhances the metabolism of pethidine and can increase pethidine clearance values by 20% and decrease pethidine AUC values by 50%.

Drug Interactions Between AEDs and Non-AED Drugs:

ANTIMICROBIALS

Antifungal agents

Griseofulvin

Phenobarbital: A decrease in the plasma level and clinical effectiveness of griseofulvin has been reported in patients taking phenobarbital. Interestingly, this interaction may not necessarily involve enzyme induction, as there is evidence that phenobarbital may impair the absorption of this antifungal.

Itraconazole

Carbamazepine: Carbamazepine enhances the metabolism of itraconazole, probably via an action on CYP3A4, and can decrease plasma itraconazole levels more than 10-fold.

Phenobarbital: The effect of phenobarbital on the pharmacokinetics of itraconazole has not been investigated but phenobarbital can be expected to have the same effect as that seen for carbamazepine and phenytoin.

Phenytoin: Phenytoin enhances the metabolism of itraconazole, probably via an action on CYP3A4, and can decrease plasma itraconazole levels more than 10-fold.

Primidone: Since primidone is metabolized to phenobarbital, primidone can be expected to affect the pharmacokinetics of itraconazole in exactly the same way as that observed with phenobarbital.

Ketoconazole

Carbamazepine: Carbamazepine enhances the metabolism of ketoconazole, probably via an action on CYP3A4, and can decrease plasma ketoconazole levels by up to 5-fold.

Phenobarbital: The effect of phenobarbital on the pharmacokinetics of ketoconazole has not been investigated but it can be expected to have the same effect as that seen for carbamazepine and phenytoin.

Phenytoin: Phenytoin enhances the metabolism of ketoconazole, probably via an action on CYP3A4, and can decrease plasma ketoconazole levels by up to 5-fold.

Primidone: Since primidone is metabolized to phenobarbital, primidone can be expected to affect the pharmacokinetics of ketoconazole in exactly the same way as that observed with phenobarbital.

Voriconazole

Phenytoin: Phenytoin enhances the metabolism of voriconazole, via an action on CYP2C9 and possibly CYP2C19, and can decrease steady-state voriconazole Cmax values by ~50% and AUC values by ~ 70%.

Anthelmintics

Albendazole

Carbamazepine: Carbamazepine enhances the metabolism of albendazole, probably via an action on CYP3A4, and can decrease albendazole AUC and elimination half-life values by 50% and can decrease plasma albendazole levels by ~ 50%.

Phenobarbital: Phenobarbital enhances the metabolism of albendazole, probably via an action on CYP3A4, and can decrease albendazole AUC values by 70% and elimination half-life values by 40% and can decrease plasma albendazole levels by ~ 65%.

Phenytoin: Phenytoin enhances the metabolism of albendazole, probably via an action on CYP3A4, and can decrease albendazole AUC values by 66% and elimination half-life values by 53% and can decrease plasma albendazole levels by ~ 65%.

Mebendazole

Carbamazepine: Carbamazepine enhances the metabolism of mebendazole and can decrease plasma mebendazole levels.

Phenytoin: Phenytoin enhances the metabolism of mebendazole and can decrease plasma mebendazole levels.

Valproic acid: Valproic acid does not affect the pharmacokinetics of mebendazole.

Drug Interactions Between AEDs and Non-AED Drugs:

Praziquantel

Carbamazepine: Carbamazepine enhances the first-pass metabolism of praziquantel and can decrease praziquantel elimination half-life values by 88% and plasma praziquantel levels by 90%.

Phenobarbital: Although the effect of phenobarbital on the metabolism of praziquantel has not been determined, a similar interaction would be expected as that described for carbamazepine and phenytoin.

Phenytoin: Phenytoin enhances the first-pass metabolism of praziquantel and can decrease praziquantel elimination half-life values by 86% and plasma praziquantel levels by 74%.

Primidone: Although the effect of primidone on the metabolism of praziquantel has not been determined, a similar interaction would be expected as that described for carbamazepine and phenytoin.

Antituberculous agents

Isoniazid

Carbamazepine: Carbamazepine enhances the metabolism of acetylhydrazine, a major metabolite of isoniazid, to a reactive intermediate thereby contributing to isoniazid-associated toxicity.

Antiviral agents

Delavirdine

Carbamazepine: Carbamazepine enhances the metabolism of delavirdine, via an action on CYP3A4, and can decrease plasma delavirdine levels.

Phenytoin: Phenytoin enhances the metabolism of delavirdine, via an action on CYP3A4, and can decrease plasma delavirdine levels.

Phenobarbital: Phenobarbital enhances the metabolism of delavirdine, via an action on CYP3A4, and can decrease plasma delavirdine levels.

Primidone: Primidone enhances the metabolism of delavirdine, via an action on CYP3A4, and can decrease plasma delavirdine levels.

Valproic acid: The effect of valproic acid on the metabolism of delavirdine has not been investigated. However, valproic acid has the potential to inhibit the metabolism of delavirdine.

Efavirenz

Carbamazepine: Carbamazepine enhances the metabolism of efavirenz, via an action on CYP3A4, and can decrease plasma efavirenz levels.

Phenytoin: Phenytoin enhances the metabolism of efavirenz, via an action on CYP3A4, and can decrease plasma efavirenz levels.

Phenobarbital: Phenobarbital enhances the metabolism of efavirenz, via an action on CYP3A4, and can decrease plasma efavirenz levels.

Primidone: Primidone enhances the metabolism of efavirenz, via an action on CYP3A4, and can decrease plasma efavirenz levels.

Valproic Acid: Valproic acid does not effect the pharmacokinetics of efavirenz.

Indinavir

Carbamazepine: Carbamazepine enhances the metabolism of indinavir, via an action on CYP3A4, and can decrease plasma indinavir levels by ~ 25%.

Phenytoin: Phenytoin enhances the metabolism of indinavir, via an action on CYP3A4, and can decrease plasma indinavir levels.

Phenobarbital: Phenobarbital enhances the metabolism of indinavir, via an action on CYP3A4, and can decrease plasma indinavir levels.

Primidone: Primidone enhances the metabolism of indinavir, via an action on CYP3A4, and can decrease plasma indinavir levels.

Lopinavir

Valproic acid Valproic acid can increase lopinavir levels.

Nelfinavir

Carbamazepine: Carbamazepine enhances the metabolism of nelfinavir, via an action on CYP3A4, and can decrease plasma nelfinavir levels.

Phenobarbital: Phenobarbital enhances the metabolism of nelfinavir, via an action on CYP3A4, and can decrease plasma nelfinavir levels.

Phenytoin: Phenytoin enhances the metabolism of nelfinavir, via an action on CYP3A4, and can decrease plasma nelfinavir levels.

Primidone: Primidone enhances the metabolism of nelfinavir, via an action on CYP3A4, and can decrease plasma nelfinavir levels.

Nevirapine

Carbamazepine: Carbamazepine enhances the metabolism of nevirapine, via an action on CYP3A4, and can decreases plasma nevirapine levels.

Phenytoin: Phenytoin enhances the metabolism of nevirapine, via an action on CYP3A4, and can decrease plasma nevirapine levels.

Phenobarbital: Phenobarbital enhances the metabolism of nevirapine, via an action on CYP3A4, and can decrease plasma nevirapine levels.

Primidone: Primidone enhances the metabolism of nevirapine, via an action on CYP3A4, and can decrease plasma nevirapine levels.

Ritonavir

Carbamazepine: Carbamazepine enhances the metabolism of ritonavir, via an action on CYP3A4, and can decrease plasma ritonavir levels.

Phenytoin: Phenytoin enhances the metabolism of ritonavir, via an action on CYP3A4, and can decrease plasma ritonavir levels.

Phenobarbital: Phenobarbital enhances the metabolism of ritonavir, via an action on CYP3A4, and can decrease plasma ritonavir levels.

Primidone: Primidone enhances the metabolism of ritonavir, via an action on CYP3A4, and can decrease plasma ritonavir levels.

Saquinavir

Carbamazepine: Carbamazepine enhances the metabolism of saquinavir, via an action on CYP3A4, and can decrease plasma saquinavir levels.

Phenytoin: Phenytoin enhances the metabolism of saquinavir, via an action on CYP3A4, and can decrease plasma saquinavir levels.

Phenobarbital: Phenobarbital enhances the metabolism of saquinavir, via an action on CYP3A4, and can decrease plasma saquinavir levels.

Primidone: Primidone enhances the metabolism of saquinavir, via an action on CYP3A4, and can decrease plasma saquinavir levels.

Valproic acid: The effect of valproic acid on the metabolism of saquinavir has not been investigated. However, valproic acid has the potential to inhibit the metabolism of saquinavir.

Zidovudine

Carbamazepine: Carbamazepine enhances the metabolism of zidovudine and can decrease plasma zidovudine levels.

Phenytoin: Phenytoin enhances the metabolism of zidovudine and can decrease plasma zidovudine levels.

Phenobarbital: Phenobarbital enhances the metabolism of zidovudine and can decrease plasma zidovudine levels.

Primidone: Primidone enhances the metabolism of zidovudine and can decrease plasma zidovudine levels.

Valproic acid: Valproic acid inhibits the metabolism of zidovudine, via an action on glucuronidation, and can increase plasma zidovudine levels 2-3-fold.

Chloramphenicol

Phenobarbital: Phenobarbital enhances the metabolism of chloramphenicol and can decrease plasma chloramphenicol levels by 70-95%.

Phenytoin: Phenytoin inhibits the metabolism of chloramphenicol and can increase chloramphenicol half-life values 2-fold and plasma chloramphenicol levels by up to 3-fold.

Fluoroquinolones

Clinafloxacin

Phenytoin: Phenytoin does not affect the pharmacokinetics of clinafloxacin.

Macrolides

Erythromycin

Carbamazepine: Carbamazepine enhances the metabolism of erythromycin, via an action on CYP3A4, and can increase the clearance of erythromycin.

Phenytoin: Phenytoin enhances the metabolism of erythromycin, via an action on CYP3A4, and can increase the clearance of erythromycin.

Metronidazole

Phenobarbital:	Phenobarbital enhances the metabolism of metronidazole.

Tetracyclines
Doxycycline

Carbamazepine:	Carbamazepine enhances the metabolism of doxycycline and can decrease the elimination half-life of doxycycline by 44%.
Phenobarbital:	Phenobarbital enhances the metabolism of doxycycline.
Phenytoin:	Phenytoin enhances the metabolism of doxycycline and can decrease the elimination half-life of doxycycline by 52%.

ANTINEOPLASTIC AGENTS

9-aminocampthotecin

Carbamazepine: Carbamazepine enhances the metabolism 9-aminocampthotecin and can decrease plasma 9-aminocampthotecin levels 3-fold.

Phenobarbital: Phenobarbital enhances the metabolism 9-aminocampthotecin and can decrease plasma 9-aminocampthotecin levels 3-fold.

Phenytoin: Phenytoin enhances the metabolism 9-aminocampthotecin and can decrease plasma 9-aminocampthotecin levels 3-fold.

Busulphan

Phenytoin: Phenytoin enhances the metabolism of busulphan and can increase busulphan clearance by $\sim$ 18%, decrease elimination half-life values by 23% and decrease AUC values by 16%.

Cisplatin

Valproic acid: Valproic acid in combination with cisplatin is associated with a 3-fold higher incidence of reversible thrombopenia, neutropenia or both. This is considered to be a consequence of a pharmacodynamic interaction and this interaction may also occur with fotemustine and etoposide.

Cyclophosphamide

Phenytoin: Phenytoin enhances the metabolism cyclophosphamide. In general, this interaction would be expected to result in decreased efficacy of cyclophosphamide. However, because the metabolism of cyclophosphamide results in a pharmacologically active metabolite, enzyme induction could theoretically potentiate drug effects by stimulating bioactivation processes. Pharmacodynamic interactions between phenytoin and cyclophosphamide may also occur.

Cytarabine

Carbamazepine: Carbamazepine does not affect the pharmacokinetics of cytarabine.

ANTINEOPLASTIC AGENTS

Phenobarbital: Phenobarbital does not affect the pharmacokinetics of cytarabine.

Phenytoin: Phenytoin does not affect the pharmacokinetics of cytarabine.

Docetaxel

Carbamazepine: Carbamazepine enhances the metabolism of docetaxel.

Phenobarbital: Phenobarbital enhances the metabolism of docetaxel.

Phenytoin: Phenytoin enhances the metabolism docetaxel.

Etoposide

Phenobarbital: Phenobarbital enhances the metabolism of etoposide and can increase etoposide clearance 2-3-fold.

Phenytoin: Phenytoin enhances the metabolism of etoposide and can increase etoposide clearance 2-3-fold.

Ifofosfamide

Phenobarbital: Phenobarbital enhances the metabolism of ifofosfamide. In general, this interaction would be expected to result in decreased efficacy of ifofosfamide. However, because the metabolism of ifofosfamide results in a pharmacologically active metabolite, enzyme induction could theoretically potentiate drug effects by stimulating bioactivation processes. Pharmacodynamic interactions between phenobarbital and ifofosfamide may also occur.

Phenytoin: Phenytoin enhances the metabolism ifofosfamide. In general, this interaction would be expected to result in decreased efficacy of ifofosfamide. However, because the metabolism of ifofosfamide results in a pharmacologically active metabolite, enzyme induction could theoretically potentiate drug effects by stimulating bioactivation processes. Pharmacodynamic interactions between phenytoin and ifofosfamide may also occur.

Irinotecan

Phenytoin: Phenytoin enhances the metabolism of irinotecan, via an action on CYP3A4, and can decrease irinotecan AUC values by ~ 60%.

Interactions Affected by AEDs

Drug Interactions Between AEDs and Non-AED Drugs:

Methotrexate

Carbamazepine: Carbamazepine enhances the metabolism of methotrexate and can increase methotrexate clearance by up to 1.5-fold.

Phenobarbital: Phenobarbital enhances the metabolism of methotrexate and can increase methotrexate clearance by up to 1.5-fold.

Phenytoin: Phenytoin enhances the metabolism of methotrexate and can increase methotrexate clearance by up to 1.5-fold.

Paclitaxel

Carbamazepine: Carbamazepine enhances the metabolism of paclitaxel and can increase paclitaxel clearance by ~ 50%.

Phenobarbital: Phenobarbital enhances the metabolism of paclitaxel and can increase paclitaxel clearance by ~ 50%.

Phenytoin: Phenytoin enhances the metabolism of paclitaxel and can increase paclitaxel clearance by ~ 50%.

Procarbazine

Carbamazepine: Carbamazepine enhances the metabolism of procarbazine and increases procarbazine hypersensitivity reactions, possibly through an intermediate generated by the induction of a CYP3A isoform.

Phenobarbital: Phenobarbital enhances the metabolism of procarbazine and increases procarbazine hypersensitivity reactions, possibly through an intermediate generated by the induction of a CYP3A isoform.

Phenytoin: Phenytoin enhances the metabolism of procarbazine and increases procarbazine hypersensitivity reactions, possibly through an intermediate generated by the induction of a CYP3A isoform.

Teniposide

Carbamazepine: Carbamazepine enhances the metabolism of teniposide, via an action on CYP3A4, and can increase teniposide clearance by up to 3-fold.

ANTINEOPLASTIC AGENTS

Phenobarbital: Phenobarbital enhances the metabolism of teniposide, via an action on CYP3A4, and can increase teniposide clearance by up to 3-fold.

Phenytoin: Phenytoin enhances the metabolism of teniposide, via an action on CYP3A4, and can increase teniposide clearance by up to 3-fold.

Topotecan

Phenytoin: Phenytoin enhances the metabolism of topotecan and can increase topotecan clearance by ~ 50%. This interaction is complicated by the fact that the plasma AUC of the N-desmethyl metabolite of topotecan, which is pharmacologically equipotent to that of topotecan, can be increased 2-fold.

Vincristine

Carbamazepine: Carbamazepine enhances the metabolism of vincristine and can increase vincristine clearance values by 63%, decrease elimination half-life values by 35% and decrease vincristine plasma AUC values by 43%.

Phenobarbital: Phenobarbital enhances the metabolism of vincristine and can increase vincristine clearance and decrease plasma vincristine levels.

Phenytoin: Phenytoin enhances the metabolism of vincristine and can increase vincristine clearance by 63% and decrease vincristine plasma AUC values by 43%.

ANTIULCER DRUGS

Proton pump inhibitors

Omeprazole

Carbamazepine: Carbamazepine enhances the metabolism of omeprazole, via an action on CYP3A4, and can decrease AUC values by 40%.

Phenobarbital: The effect of phenobarbital on omeprazole pharmacokinetics is not known. However, the potential exists for phenobarbital to enhance the metabolism of omeprazole by an action on CYP2C19 and CYP3A4.

Phenytoin: The effect of phenytoin on omeprazole pharmacokinetics is not known. However, the potential exists for phenytoin to enhance the metabolism of omeprazole by an action on CYP2C19 and CYP3A4.

Drug Interactions Between AEDs and Non-AED Drugs:

CARDIOVASCULAR DRUGS

Antiarrhythmics

Amiodarone

Carbamazepine: Carbamazepine enhances the metabolism of amiodarone and can decrease plasma amiodarone levels.

Phenytoin: Phenytoin enhances the metabolism of amiodarone and can decrease plasma amiodarone levels by 20-55%.

Disopyramide

Phenytoin: Phenytoin enhances the metabolism of disopyramide and can increase disopyramide clearance 2.5-fold, decrease disopyramide AUC values by 54% and decrease disopyramide elimination half-life values by 62%. That there is a concurrent 2.7-fold increase in the AUC values of the pharmacologically active metabolite (mono-N-dealkyldisopyramide) of disopyramide, complicates the interpretation of this interaction.

Mexiletine

Phenytoin: Phenytoin enhances the metabolism of mexiletine and can decrease mexiletine AUC values by ~55% and decrease mexiletine elimination half-life values by ~50%.

Quinidine

Phenobarbital: Phenobarbital enhances the metabolism of quinidine and can decrease quinidine elimination half-life values by ~60% and increase quinidine clearance values by ~60%.

Phenytoin: Phenytoin enhances the metabolism of quinidine and can decrease quinidine elimination half-life values by ~60% and increase quinidine clearance values by ~60%.

Antihypertensive agents

Alprenolol

Phenobarbital: Phenobarbital enhances the metabolism of alprenolol and can decrease plasma alprenolol levels by 50%.

Atenolol

Phenobarbital: Phenobarbital does not affect the pharmacokinetics of atenolol.

Felodipine

Carbamazepine: Carbamazepine enhances the metabolism of felodipine and can decrease felodipine AUC values by 94% and plasma felodipine levels by 80-95%.

Phenobarbital: Phenobarbital enhances the metabolism of felodipine and can decrease felodipine AUC values by 94% and plasma felodipine levels by 80-95%.

Phenytoin: Phenytoin enhances the metabolism of felodipine and can decrease felodipine AUC values by 94% and plasma felodipine levels by 80-95%.

Oxcarbazepine: Oxcarbazepine enhances the metabolism of felodipine and can decrease felodipine Cmax values by 34% and AUC values by 28%.

Losartan

Phenytoin: Whilst phenytoin has no effect on plasma losartan levels, phenytoin can decrease plasma levels of the pharmacologically active carboxylic acid metabolite (E3174) of losartan by 63%. The mechanism of the interaction is via an inhibition of CYP2C9-mediated formation clearance. Therefore, a reduced antihypertensive effect may be anticipated.

Drug Interactions Between AEDs and Non-AED Drugs:

Nadolol
Phenobarbital: Phenobarbital does not affect the pharmacokinetics of nadolol.

Nifedipine
Carbamazepine: Carbamazepine can be expected to enhance the metabolism of nifedipine.

Phenobarbital: Phenobarbital enhances the metabolism of nifedipine and can decrease nifedipine AUC values by 60%.

Phenytoin: Phenytoin can be expected to enhance the metabolism of nifedipine.

Nimodipine
Carbamazepine: Carbamazepine enhances the metabolism of nimodipine and can decrease nimodipine AUC values 7-fold and plasma nimodipine levels by 8-10-fold.

Phenobarbital: Phenobarbital enhances the metabolism of nimodipine and can decrease nimodipine AUC values 7-fold and plasma nimodipine levels by 8-10-fold.

Phenytoin: Phenytoin enhances the metabolism of nimodipine and can decrease nimodipine AUC values 7-fold and plasma nimodipine levels by 8-10-fold.

Valproic acid: Valproic acid inhibits the metabolism of nimodipine and can increase plasma nimodipine levels by 50%.

Nisoldipine
Phenytoin: Phenytoin enhances the metabolism of nisoldipine and can decrease nisoldipine AUC values by ~10-fold.

Nivadipine
Carbamazepine: Carbamazepine enhances the metabolism of nivadipine, probably via an action on CYP3A4, and can decrease plasma nivadipine levels.

Propranolol

Carbamazepine: Carbamazepine can be expected to enhance the metabolism of propranolol.

Phenobarbital: Phenobarbital enhances the metabolism of propranolol and can decrease plasma propranolol levels.

Phenytoin: Phenytoin can be expected to enhance the metabolism of propranolol.

Topiramate: Topiramate decreases the clearance of propranolol by 9% and can increase plasma propranolol levels by 10% and plasma 4-hydroxy-propranolol (the pharmacologically active metabolite of propranolol) by 17%.

Sotalol

Phenobarbital: Phenobarbital does not affect the pharmacokinetics of sotalol.

Verapamil

Carbamazepine: Carbamazepine inhibits the metabolism of verapamil and can increase plasma verapamil levels by 40%.

Phenobarbital: Phenobarbital enhances the metabolism of verapamil and can increase verapamil clearance 4-fold and decrease plasma verapamil levels 5-fold.

Phenytoin: Phenytoin enhances the metabolism of verapamil.

Digoxin

Levetiracetam: Levetiracetam does not affect the pharmacokinetics of digoxin.

Phenytoin: Phenytoin enhances the metabolism of digoxin and can decrease elimination half-life values by 30%, decrease AUC values by 23% and decrease plasma digoxin levels by 22%.

Tiagabine: Tiagabine does not affect the pharmacokinetics of digoxin.

Topiramate: Topiramate (200 mg/day) can increase digoxin clearance by 13%.

Drug Interactions Between AEDs and Non-AED Drugs:

Diuretics
Furosemide (frusemide)

Phenytoin: Phenytoin delays and reduces the magnitude of the diuretic effect of furosemide. It is thought that the mechanism of this interaction is a phenytoin-induced decrease in the spontaneous activity of gastrointestinal smooth muscle leading to reduced furosemide absorption. Additionally, a pharmacodynamic interaction might occur since renal responsiveness to furosemide is also impaired.

Oral anticoagulants
Dicoumarol

Carbamazepine: Carbamazepine enhances the metabolism of dicoumarol, possibly via an action on CYP2C9, and can reduce the anticoagulant effects of dicoumarol.

Phenobarbital: Phenobarbital enhances the metabolism of dicoumarol, possibly via an action on CYP2C9, and can reduce the anticoagulant effects of dicoumarol.

Phenytoin: Phenytoin enhances the metabolism of dicoumarol, possibly via an action on CYP2C9, and can reduce the anticoagulant effects of dicoumarol.

Primidone: Primidone enhances the metabolism of dicoumarol, possibly via an action on CYP2C9, and can reduce the anticoagulant effects of dicoumarol.

Phenprocoumon

Carbamazepine: Carbamazepine reduces the anticoagulant effects of phenprocoumon, possibly by increasing its metabolism.

Valproic acid: Valproic acid does not affect the anticoagulant effect of phenprocoumon.

Warfarin

Carbamazepine: Carbamazepine enhances the metabolism of warfarin resulting in a reduction in warfarin elimination half-life values and a decrease in plasma warfarin levels and a decrease in the prothrombin time response to warfarin. Typically, a 2-fold increase in warfarin dosage is required so as to maintain an appropriate international normalized ratio (INR). Because enzyme induction may take several weeks to fully develop or subside, frequent monitoring of INR with appropriate dosage adjustment is advised for at least 4 weeks after starting or stopping carbamazepine.

Felbamate: Felbamate inhibits the metabolism of warfarin resulting in an increased INR.

Levetiracetam: Levetiracetam (2000 mg/day) does not affect the pharmacokinetics of warfarin.

Oxcarbazepine: Oxcarbazepine (900 mg/day) does not affect the pharmacokinetics of warfarin.

Phenobarbital: Phenobarbital enhances the metabolism of warfarin and decreases the prothrombin time response to warfarin. Typically, a 25%-50% increase in warfarin dosage is required. Because enzyme induction may take several weeks to fully develop or subside, frequent monitoring of INR with appropriate dosage adjustment is advised for at least 4 weeks after starting or stopping phenobarbital.

Phenytoin: Despite an expected induction of warfarin metabolism by phenytoin, several cases of hypoprothrombinemia and severe bleeding complications have been reported after addition of phenytoin to warfarin. Proposed mechanisms for an enhanced anticoagulant response are displacement of warfarin from plasma protein binding sites or inhibition of its metabolism by phenytoin.

Because of potential induction and inhibition of warfarin metabolism via CYP2C9 by phenytoin, the occurrence of a biphasic interaction has been suggested, with warfarin plasma levels initially increasing due to inhibition and then decreasing after 1-2 weeks as enzyme induction predominates.

Due to the unpredictability of this interaction, frequent monitoring of INR with appropriate dosage adjustment is advised for at least 4 weeks after starting or stopping phenytoin.

Thus, the interaction between phenytoin and warfarin is complex in that after an initial enhancement in anticoagulant action, the latter can be subsequently decreased.

Tiagabine: Tiagabine (12 mg/day) does not affect the pharmacokinetics of warfarin.

IMMUNOSUPPRESSANTS

Cyclosporin A

Carbamazepine: Carbamazepine enhances the metabolism of cyclosporine, via an action on CYP3A4, and can decrease plasma cyclosporine levels.

Ethosuximide: Ethosuximide does not affect the pharmacokinetics of cyclosporin.

Oxcarbazepine: Oxcarbazepine can decrease plasma cyclosporin levels by up to 25%.

Phenobarbital: Phenobarbital enhances the metabolism of cyclosporin, via an action on CYP3A4, and can decrease plasma cyclosporin levels by more than 50%.

Phenytoin: Phenytoin enhances the metabolism of cyclosporin, via an action on CYP3A4, and can decrease plasma cyclosporin levels by more than 40%.

Primidone: Primidone enhances the metabolism of cyclosporin, via an action on CYP3A4, and can decrease plasma cyclosporin levels.

Valproic acid: Valproic acid does not affect the pharmacokinetics of cyclosporin. However its use, particularly in renal transplant recipients, should be weighed out against possible risks of hepatotoxicity consequent to its metabolite(s).

Tacrolimus

Phenytoin: Phenytoin enhances the metabolism of tacrolimus, via induction of CYP3A, and can decrease plasma tacrolimus levels. The interaction may be bi-directional in that tacrolimus can also inhibit the metabolism of phenytoin.

Sirolimus

Phenytoin: Phenytoin enhances the metabolism of sirolimus, via an action on CYP3A4/5, and can increase sirolimus clearance by up to 4-fold and decrease plasma sirolimus levels.

NEUROMUSCULAR BLOCKING AGENTS

Atracurium

Carbamazepine: Carbamazepine does not affect the pharmacokinetics of atracurium.

Phenytoin: Phenytoin does not affect the pharmacokinetics of atracurium.

Cisatracurium

Carbamazepine: Carbamazepine enhances the metabolism of cisatracurium. Patients receiving chronic therapy with carbamazepine show a decreased duration of neuromuscular blockade and higher cisatracurium dosage requirements. Both pharmacokinetic (enzyme induction) and pharmacodynamic (upregulation of acetylcholine receptors) mechanisms may explain this interaction.

Phenytoin: Phenytoin enhances the metabolism of cisatracurium. Patients receiving chronic therapy with phenytoin show a decreased duration of neuromuscular blockade and higher cisatracurium dosage requirements. Both pharmacokinetic (enzyme induction) and pharmacodynamic (upregulation of acetylcholine receptors) mechanisms may explain this interaction.

Doxacurium

Carbamazepine: Carbamazepine enhances the metabolism of doxacurium. Patients receiving chronic therapy with carbamazepine show a decreased duration of neuromuscular blockade and higher doxacurium dosage requirements. Both pharmacokinetic (enzyme induction) and pharmacodynamic (upregulation of acetylcholine receptors) mechanisms may explain this interaction.

Phenytoin: Phenytoin enhances the metabolism of doxacurium. Patients receiving chronic therapy with phenytoin show a decreased duration of neuromuscular blockade and higher doxacurium dosage requirements. Both pharmacokinetic (enzyme induction) and pharmacodynamic (upregulation of acetylcholine receptors) mechanisms may explain this interaction.

Mivacurium

Carbamazepine: Carbamazepine does not affect the pharmacokinetics of mivacurium.

Phenytoin: Phenytoin does not affect the pharmacokinetics of mivacurium.

Valproic acid: Valproic acid does not affect the pharmacokinetics of mivacurium.

Pancuronium

Carbamazepine: Carbamazepine enhances the metabolism of pancuronium. Patients receiving chronic therapy with carbamazepine show a decreased duration of neuromuscular blockade and higher pancuronium dosage requirements. Both pharmacokinetic (enzyme induction) and pharmacodynamic (upregulation of acetylcholine receptors) mechanisms may explain this interaction.

Phenytoin: Phenytoin enhances the metabolism of pancuronium. Patients receiving chronic therapy with phenytoin show a decreased duration of neuromuscular blockade and higher pancuronium dosage requirements. Both pharmacokinetic (enzyme induction) and pharmacodynamic (upregulation of acetylcholine receptors) mechanisms may explain this interaction.

Rapacuronium

Carbamazepine: Carbamazepine enhances the metabolism of rapacuronium. Patients receiving chronic therapy with carbamazepine show a decreased duration of neuromuscular blockade and higher rapacuronium dosage requirements. Both pharmacokinetic (enzyme induction) and pharmacodynamic (upregulation of acetylcholine receptors) mechanisms may explain this interaction.

Phenytoin: Phenytoin enhances the metabolism of rapacuronium. Patients receiving chronic therapy with phenytoin show a decreased duration of neuromuscular blockade and higher rapacuronium dosage requirements. Both pharmacokinetic (enzyme induction) and pharmacodynamic (upregulation of acetylcholine receptors) mechanisms may explain this interaction.

Rocuronium

Carbamazepine: Carbamazepine enhances the metabolism of rocuronium. Patients receiving chronic therapy with carbamazepine show a decreased duration of neuromuscular blockade and higher rocuronium dosage requirements. Both pharmacokinetic (enzyme induction) and pharmacodynamic (upregulation of acetylcholine receptors) mechanisms may explain this interaction.

Phenytoin: Phenytoin does not affect the pharmacokinetics of rocuronium when administered acutely. However, when administered chronically, phenytoin enhances the metabolism of rocuronium. Patients receiving chronic therapy with phenytoin show a decreased duration of neuromuscular blockade and higher rocuronium dosage requirements. Both pharmacokinetic (enzyme induction) and pharmacodynamic (upregulation of acetylcholine receptors) mechanisms may explain this interaction.

Primidone: Primidone enhances the metabolism of rocuronium. Patients receiving chronic therapy with primidone show a decreased duration of neuromuscular blockade and higher rocuronium dosage requirements. Both pharmacokinetic (enzyme induction) and pharmacodynamic (upregulation of acetylcholine receptors) mechanisms may explain this interaction.

Vecuronium

Carbamazepine: Carbamazepine enhances the metabolism of vecuronium and can decrease vecuronium elimination half-life values by 62% and can increase vecuronium clearance values 2-fold. Patients receiving chronic therapy with carbamazepine show a decreased duration of neuromuscular blockade and higher vecuronium dosage requirements. Both pharmacokinetic (enzyme induction) and pharmacodynamic (upregulation of acetylcholine receptors) mechanisms may explain this interaction.

Phenytoin: Phenytoin enhances the metabolism of vecuronium and can decrease vecuronium elimination half-life values by 51% and can increase vecuronium clearance values by 68%. Patients receiving chronic therapy with phenytoin show a decreased duration of neuromuscular blockade and higher vecuronium dosage requirements. Both pharmacokinetic (enzyme induction) and pharmacodynamic (upregulation of acetylcholine receptors) mechanisms may explain this interaction.

PSYCHOTROPIC DRUGS

Antidepressants

Amitriptyline

Carbamazepine: Carbamazepine enhances the metabolism of amitriptyline and can decrease plasma amitriptyline levels.

Phenobarbital: Phenobarbital enhances the metabolism of amitriptyline and can decrease plasma amitriptyline levels.

Phenytoin: Phenytoin enhances the metabolism of amitriptyline and can decrease plasma amitriptyline levels.

Primidone: Primidone enhances the metabolism of amitriptyline and can decrease plasma amitriptyline levels.

Topiramate: Topiramate can increase mean plasma amitriptyline and nortriptyline (the pharmacologically active metabolite of amitriptyline) levels by 8% and 19% respectively.

Valproic acid: Valproic acid inhibits the metabolism of amitriptyline and can increase plasma amitriptyline levels by 50-60%.

Citalopram

Carbamazepine: Carbamazepine enhances the metabolism of citalopram, probably via an action on CYP3A4, and can decrease citalopram plasma levels by 30%.

Phenobarbital: Phenobarbital enhances the metabolism of citalopram and can decrease plasma citalopram levels.

Phenytoin: Phenytoin enhances the metabolism of citalopram and can decrease plasma citalopram levels.

Primidone: Primidone enhances the metabolism of citalopram and can decrease plasma citalopram levels.

Clomipramine

Carbamazepine: Carbamazepine enhances the metabolism of clomipramine and can decrease plasma clomipramine levels.

Phenobarbital: Phenobarbital enhances the metabolism of clomipramine and can decrease plasma clomipramine levels.

Phenytoin:	Phenytoin enhances the metabolism of clomipramine and can decrease plasma clomipramine levels.
Primidone:	Primidone enhances the metabolism of clomipramine and can decrease plasma clomipramine levels.
Valproic acid:	Valproic acid inhibits the metabolism of clomipramine and can increase plasma clomipramine levels.

Desipramine

Carbamazepine:	Carbamazepine enhances the metabolism of desipramine and can decrease plasma desipramine levels.
Phenobarbital:	Phenobarbital enhances the metabolism of desipramine and can decrease plasma desipramine levels.
Phenytoin:	Phenytoin enhances the metabolism of desipramine and can decrease plasma desipramine levels.
Primidone:	Primidone enhances the metabolism of desipramine and can decrease plasma desipramine levels.

Desmethylclomipramine

Carbamazepine:	Carbamazepine enhances the metabolism of desmethylclomipramine and can decrease plasma desmethylclomipramine levels.
Phenobarbital:	Phenobarbital enhances the metabolism of desmethylclomipramine and can decrease plasma desmethylclomipramine levels.
Phenytoin:	Phenytoin enhances the metabolism of desmethylclomipramine and can decrease plasma desmethylclomipramine levels.
Primidone:	Primidone enhances the metabolism of desmethylclomipramine and can decrease plasma desmethylclomipramine levels.

Doxepin

Carbamazepine:	Carbamazepine enhances the metabolism of doxepin and can decrease plasma doxepin levels by 50%.

Drug Interactions Between AEDs and Non-AED Drugs:

Phenobarbital: Phenobarbital can be expected to enhance the metabolism of doxepin and to decrease plasma doxepin levels.

Phenytoin: Phenytoin can be expected to enhance the metabolism of doxepin and to decrease plasma doxepin levels.

Primidone: Primidone can be expected to enhance the metabolism of doxepin and to decrease plasma doxepin levels.

Fluoxetine

Carbamazepine: Carbamazepine appears not to affect the pharmacokinetics of fluoxetine. However, a pharmacodynamic interaction (toxic serotonin syndrome) can occur between the two drugs.

Imipramine

Carbamazepine: Carbamazepine enhances the metabolism of imipramine and can decrease plasma imipramine levels by 42%.

Phenobarbital: Phenobarbital enhances the metabolism of imipramine and can decrease plasma imipramine levels.

Phenytoin: Phenytoin enhances the metabolism of imipramine and can decrease plasma imipramine levels.

Primidone: Primidone enhances the metabolism of imipramine and can decrease plasma imipramine levels.

Mianserin

Carbamazepine: Carbamazepine enhances the metabolism of mianserin and can decrease plasma mianserin levels by 70%.

Phenobarbital: Phenobarbital enhances the metabolism of mianserin and can decrease plasma mianserin levels.

Phenytoin: Phenytoin enhances the metabolism of mianserin and can decrease plasma mianserin levels.

Mirtazapine

Carbamazepine: Carbamazepine enhances the metabolism of mirtazapine and can increase mirtazapine clearance values 2.5-fold and can decrease mirtazapine AUC values and plasma mirtazapine levels by 61%.

Phenytoin:	Phenytoin enhances the metabolism of mirtazapine and can decrease mirtazapine AUC values by 47% and plasma mirtazapine levels by 33%.

Nefazodone

Carbamazepine:	Carbamazepine enhances the metabolism of nefazodone and can decrease AUC values by 92%.
Phenobarbital:	Phenobarbital enhances the metabolism of nefazodone and can decrease plasma nefazodone levels.
Phenytoin:	Phenytoin enhances the metabolism of nefazodone and can decrease plasma nefazodone levels.
Primidone:	Primidone enhances the metabolism of nefazodone and can decrease plasma nefazodone levels.

Nortriptyline

Carbamazepine:	Carbamazepine enhances the metabolism of nortriptyline and can decrease plasma nortriptyline levels.
Phenobarbital:	Phenobarbital enhances the metabolism of nortriptyline and can decrease plasma nortriptyline levels.
Phenytoin:	Phenytoin enhances the metabolism of nortriptyline and can decrease plasma nortriptyline levels.
Primidone:	Primidone enhances the metabolism of nortriptyline and can decrease plasma nortriptyline levels.
Valproic acid:	Valproic acid inhibits the metabolism of nortriptyline and can increase plasma nortriptyline levels by 50-60%.

Paroxetine

Carbamazepine:	Carbamazepine enhances the metabolism of paroxetine and can decrease plasma paroxetine levels.
Lamotrigine:	Lamotrigine does not affect the pharmacokinetics of paroxetine.
Phenobarbital:	Phenobarbital enhances the metabolism of paroxetine and can decrease plasma paroxetine levels by 25%.
Phenytoin:	Phenytoin enhances the metabolism of paroxetine and can decrease plasma paroxetine levels by 50%.

Drug Interactions Between AEDs and Non-AED Drugs:

Primidone: Primidone enhances the metabolism of paroxetine and can decrease plasma paroxetine levels.

Valproic acid: Valproic acid inhibits the metabolism of paroxetine and can increase plasma paroxetine levels.

Protriptyline
Carbamazepine: Carbamazepine enhances the metabolism of protriptyline and can decrease plasma protriptyline levels.

Phenobarbital: Phenobarbital enhances the metabolism of protriptyline and can decrease plasma protriptyline levels.

Phenytoin: Phenytoin enhances the metabolism of protriptyline and can decrease plasma protriptyline levels.

Primidone: Primidone enhances the metabolism of protriptyline and can decrease plasma protriptyline levels.

Sertraline
Carbamazepine: Carbamazepine enhances the metabolism of sertraline and can decrease plasma sertraline levels. However, plasma levels of its metabolite, desmethylsertraline, are increased concurrently.

Viloxazine
Carbamazepine: Carbamazepine does not affect the pharmacokinetics of viloxazine.

Phenobarbital: Phenobarbital does not affect the pharmacokinetics of viloxazine.

Phenytoin: Phenytoin does not affect the pharmacokinetics of viloxazine.

Antipsychotics
Aripiprazole
Valproic acid: Valproic acid inhibits the metabolism of aripiprazole and can increase aripiprazole AUC and Cmax values by 24% and 25% respectively.

Clozapine

Carbamazepine: Carbamazepine enhances the metabolism of clozapine and can decrease plasma clozapine levels by 31-63%. Combining carbamazepine with clozapine is generally contraindicated due to concerns about potential additive adverse haematological side effects.

Phenytoin: Phenytoin enhances the metabolism of clozapine and can decrease plasma clozapine levels by 75-84%.

Phenobarbital: Phenobarbital enhances the metabolism of clozapine, via the enhancement of N-oxidation and demethylation pathways, and can decrease plasma clozapine levels by ~ 35%.

Primidone: The effect of primidone on the pharmacokinetics of clozapine has not been investigated. Nevertheless, primidone can be expected to interact with clozapine in a similar manner to that described for phenobarbital.

Valproic acid: There are conflicting reports on the potential effects of valproic acid on plasma clozapine levels. One study observed a 57% increase in plasma clozapine levels with the addition of valproic acid; while a second study found a 15% decrease. Both studies observed a decrease in plasma levels of norclozapine, the demethylated metabolite of clozapine. A third study reported a 41% decrease in plasma clozapine levels.

Chlorpromazine

Phenobarbital: Phenobarbital enhances the metabolism of chlorpromazine and can decrease plasma chlorpromazine levels by ~25%.

Valproic acid: Valproic acid inhibits the metabolism of chlorpromazine and can increase plasma chlorpromazine levels by ~ 20%.

Fluphenazine

Carbamazepine: Carbamazepine enhances the metabolism of fluphenazine and can decrease plasma fluphenazine levels by 49%.

Phenobarbital: Phenobarbital enhances the metabolism of fluphenazine and can decrease plasma fluphenazine levels.

Drug Interactions Between AEDs and Non-AED Drugs:

Phenytoin: Phenytoin enhances the metabolism of fluphenazine and can decrease plasma fluphenazine levels.

Primidone: Primidone via its metabolite, phenobarbital, enhances the metabolism of fluphenazine and can decrease plasma fluphenazine levels.

Haloperidol

Carbamazepine: Carbamazepine enhances the metabolism of haloperidol and can decrease plasma haloperidol levels by 34-47%.

Phenobarbital: Phenobarbital enhances the metabolism of haloperidol and can decrease plasma haloperidol levels by 50-60%.

Phenytoin: Phenytoin enhances the metabolism of haloperidol and can decrease plasma haloperidol levels by 50-60%.

Primidone: Primidone via its metabolite, phenobarbital, enhances the metabolism of haloperidol and can decrease plasma haloperidol levels by 50-60%.

Topiramate: Topiramate (200mg/day) can increase plasma haloperidol AUC values by up to 28%. The AUC values of the pharmacologically active metabolite of haloperidol are concurrently increased by up to 50%.

Valproic acid: Valproic acid does not affect the pharmacokinetics of haloperidol.

Olanzapine

Carbamazepine: Carbamazepine enhances the metabolism of olanzapine and can increase olanzapine clearance by 18% and can decrease plasma olanzapine levels by 25%.

Phenobarbital: Phenobarbital enhances the metabolism of olanzapine and can decrease plasma olanzapine levels.

Phenytoin: Phenytoin enhances the metabolism of olanzapine and can decrease plasma olanzapine levels.

Primidone: Primidone via its metabolite, phenobarbital, can enhance the metabolism of olanzapine and can decrease plasma olanzapine levels.

Valproic acid:	Valproic acid does not affect the pharmacokinetics of olanzapine.

Quetiapine

Carbamazepine:	Carbamazepine enhances the metabolism of quetiapine and can decrease plasma quetiapine levels.
Phenobarbital:	Phenobarbital enhances the metabolism of quetiapine and can decrease plasma quetiapine levels.
Phenytoin:	Phenytoin enhances the metabolism of quetiapine, probably via an action on CYP3A4, and can increase quetiapine clearance 5-fold.
Primidone:	Primidone, via its metabolite phenobarbital, enhances the metabolism of quetiapine and can decrease plasma quetiapine levels.

Risperidone

Carbamazepine:	Carbamazepine enhances the metabolism of risperidone and its pharmacologically active metabolite 9-OH-risperidone, probably via an action on CYP3A4, and can decrease plasma risperidone and 9-OH-risperidone levels by 68% and 64% respectively.
Phenobarbital:	Phenobarbital enhances the metabolism of risperidone and can decrease plasma risperidone levels.
Phenytoin:	Phenytoin enhances the metabolism of risperidone and can decrease plasma risperidone levels.
Primidone:	Primidone enhances the metabolism of risperidone and can decrease plasma risperidone levels.
Topiramate:	Topiramate (200mg/day) can decrease mean plasma risperidone AUC values by 24% and plasma levels by 29%. Mean 5-hydroxy-risperidone (the pharmacologically active metabolite of risperidone) AUC values are concurrently decreased by 8% and plasma levels by 12%.
Valproic acid:	Valproic acid does not affect the pharmacokinetics of risperidone.

Thioridazine

Carbamazepine: Carbamazepine enhances the metabolism of thioridazine and can decrease plasma thioridazine levels by 10%. However, carbamazepine also enhances the metabolism of the pharmacologically active metabolite of thioridazine (mesoridazine) and can decrease plasma mesoridazine levels by 25%.

Phenytoin: Phenytoin enhances the metabolism of thioridazine and can decrease plasma thioridazine levels by 10%. However, phenytoin also enhances the metabolism of the pharmacologically active metabolite of thioridazine (mesoridazine) and can decrease plasma mesoridazine levels by 25%.

Phenobarbital: The effect of phenobarbital on the pharmacokinetics of thioridazine has not been investigated. Nevertheless, it can be expected that phenobarbital will interact in a similar manner to that described for carbamazepine and phenytoin.

Primidone: The effect of primidone on the pharmacokinetics of thioridazine has not been investigated. Nevertheless, it can be expected that primidone, via its metabolite phenobarbital, will interact in a similar manner to that described for carbamazepine and phenytoin.

Ziprasidone

Carbamazepine: Carbamazepine enhances the metabolism of ziprasidone and can decrease ziprasidone AUC values by 36% and plasma ziprasidone levels by 27%.

Phenobarbital: Phenobarbital enhances the metabolism of ziprasidone and can decrease plasma ziprasidone levels.

Phenytoin: Phenytoin enhances the metabolism of ziprasidone and can decrease plasma ziprasidone levels.

Primidone: Primidone enhances the metabolism of ziprasidone and can decrease plasma ziprasidone levels.

Benzodiazepines

Alprazolam

Carbamazepine: Carbamazepine enhances the metabolism of alprazolam and can decrease plasma alprazolam levels.

Phenobarbital: Phenobarbital enhances the metabolism of alprazolam and can decrease plasma alprazolam levels.

Phenytoin: Phenytoin enhances the metabolism of alprazolam and can decrease plasma alprazolam levels.

Primidone: Primidone enhances the metabolism of alprazolam and can decrease plasma alprazolam levels.

Clobazam

Carbamazepine: Carbamazepine enhances the metabolism of clobazam. Typically, plasma levels of the pharmacologically active metabolite of clobazam, N-desmethylclobazam, are increased during co-medication and the blood level to weight-adjusted dose ratio of N-desmethylclobazam and clobazam can be expected to be 2-fold higher and 2-fold lower respectively.

Felbamate: Felbamate inhibits the metabolism of clobazam. Plasma levels of the pharmacologically active metabolite of clobazam, N-desmethylclobazam, are increased during co-medication with felbamate. Typically, the plasma level to weight-adjusted dose ratio of N-desmethylclobazam and clobazam can be expected to be 5-fold lower and 2-fold higher respectively. The interaction may be the consequence of inhibition of N-desmethylclobazam metabolism through CYP2C19.

Lamotrigine: Lamotrigine does not affect the pharmacokinetics of clobazam.

Levetiracetam: Levetiracetam does not affect the pharmacokinetics of clobazam.

Phenobarbital: Phenobarbital enhances the metabolism of clobazam. Typically, plasma levels of the pharmacologically active metabolite of clobazam, N-desmethylclobazam, are increased during co-medication and the blood level to weight-adjusted dose ratio of N-desmethylclobazam and clobazam can be expected to be 2-fold higher and 2-fold lower respectively.

Drug Interactions Between AEDs and Non-AED Drugs:

Phenytoin: Phenytoin enhances the metabolism of clobazam. Typically, plasma levels of the pharmacologically active metabolite of clobazam, N-desmethylclobazam, are increased during co-medication and the blood level to weight-adjusted dose ratio of N-desmethylclobazam and clobazam can be expected to be 2-fold higher and 2-fold lower respectively.

Primidone: Primidone enhances the metabolism of clobazam. Typically, plasma levels of the pharmacologically active metabolite of clobazam, N-desmethylclobazam, are increased during co-medication and the blood level to weight-adjusted dose ratio of N-desmethylclobazam and clobazam can be expected to be 2-fold higher and 2-fold lower respectively.

Clonazepam

Carbamazepine: Carbamazepine enhances the metabolism of clonazepam and can decrease plasma clonazepam levels by 19-37%.

Felbamate: Felbamate does not affect the pharmacokinetics of clonazepam.

Lamotrigine: Lamotrigine enhances the metabolism of clonazepam and can decrease plasma clonazepam levels by 20-38%.

Phenobarbital: Phenobarbital enhances the metabolism of clonazepam and can decrease plasma clonazepam levels by 19-24%.

Phenytoin: Phenytoin enhances the metabolism of clonazepam and can decrease plasma clonazepam levels by 46-58%.

Diazepam

Carbamazepine: Carbamazepine enhances the metabolism of N-desmethyldiazepam (the pharmacologically active metabolite of diazepam) and can decrease plasma N-desmethyldiazepam levels.

Phenobarbital: Phenobarbital enhances the metabolism of N-desmethyldiazepam (the pharmacologically active metabolite of diazepam) and can decrease plasma N-desmethyldiazepam levels.

Phenytoin: Phenytoin enhances the metabolism of N-desmethyldiazepam (the pharmacologically active metabolite of diazepam) and can decrease plasma N-desmethyldiazepam levels.

Primidone:	Primidone enhances the metabolism of N-desmethyldiazepam (the pharmacologically active metabolite of diazepam) and can decrease plasma N-desmethyldiazepam levels.
Valproic acid:	Valproic acid displaces diazepam from its plasma protein binding (albumin) sites. The consequence of this interaction is that the effect of intravenous diazepam may be transiently potentiated.

Lorazepam

Valproic acid:	Valproic acid can increase plasma lorazepam levels by ~ 20%.
Pregabalin:	Pregabalin does not affect the pharmacokinetics of lorazepam. However, during combination therapy impairment of cognitive and gross motor functions are observed and these are considered to be the consequence of a pharmacodynamic interaction.

Midazolam

Carbamazepine:	Carbamazepine enhances the metabolism of midazolam and can decrease plasma midazolam levels. Because the decrease in plasma levels of orally administered midazolam in patients taking carbamazepine is so marked (95%), the loss of efficacy of the hypnotic can be readily anticipated. However, since midazolam clearance after intravenous administration is more dependent on liver blood flow than on enzyme activity, this interaction would be expected to be far less important when midazolam is given parenterally.
Phenobarbital:	Phenobarbital enhances the metabolism of midazolam and can decrease plasma midazolam levels. Because the decrease in plasma levels of orally administered midazolam in patients taking phenobarbital is so marked (95%), the loss of efficacy of the hypnotic can be readily anticipated. However, since midazolam clearance after intravenous administration is more dependent on liver blood flow than on enzyme activity, this interaction would be expected to be far less important when midazolam is given parenterally.

Drug Interactions Between AEDs and Non-AED Drugs:

Phenytoin: Phenytoin enhances the metabolism of midazolam and can decrease plasma midazolam levels. Because the decrease in plasma levels of orally administered midazolam in patients taking phenytoin is so marked (95%), the loss of efficacy of the hypnotic can be readily anticipated. However, since midazolam clearance after intravenous administration is more dependent on liver blood flow than on enzyme activity, this interaction would be expected to be far less important when midazolam is given parenterally.

Primidone: Primidone enhances the metabolism of midazolam and can decrease plasma midazolam levels. Because the decrease in plasma levels of orally administered midazolam in patients taking primidone is so marked (95%), the loss of efficacy of the hypnotic can be readily anticipated. However, since midazolam clearance after intravenous administration is more dependent on liver blood flow than on enzyme activity, this interaction would be expected to be far less important when midazolam is given parenterally.

Lithium

Carbamazepine: Carbamazepine does not affect the pharmacokinetics of lithium. However, a pharmacodynamic interaction, leading to neurotoxic symptoms in patients receiving lithium in combination with carbamazepine has been reported.

Clonazepam: Clonazepam can increase plasma lithium levels by 33-61%.

Gabapentin: Gabapentin does not affect the pharmacokinetics of lithium.

Lamotrigine: Lamotrigine does not affect the pharmacokinetics of lithium.

Topiramate: Topiramate can decrease plasma lithium levels by 11-16%. This may be the consequence of carbonic anhydrase inhibition by topiramate.

Valproic acid: Valproic acid does not affect the pharmacokinetics of lithium. However, a pharmacodynamic interaction, leading to neurotoxic symptoms in patients receiving lithium in combination with valproic acid has been reported.

STEROIDS

Corticosteroids
Cortisol

Carbamazepine: Carbamazepine enhances the metabolism of cortisol and can decrease plasma cortisol levels.

Phenobarbital: Phenobarbital enhances the metabolism of cortisol and can decrease plasma cortisol levels.

Phenytoin: Phenytoin enhances the metabolism of cortisol and can decrease plasma cortisol levels.

Dexamethasone

Carbamazepine: Carbamazepine enhances the metabolism of dexamethasone and can increase dexamethasone clearance 2-4-fold.

Phenobarbital: Phenobarbital enhances the metabolism of dexamethasone and can increase dexamethasone clearance.

Phenytoin: Phenytoin enhances the metabolism of dexamethasone and can decrease dexamethasone elimination half-life values by ~ 50% and can increase dexamethasone clearance 2-fold.

Hydrocortisone

Carbamazepine: Carbamazepine enhances the metabolism of hydrocortisone and can decrease plasma hydrocortisone levels.

Phenobarbital: Phenobarbital enhances the metabolism of hydrocortisone and can decrease plasma hydrocortisone levels.

Phenytoin: Phenytoin enhances the metabolism of hydrocortisone and can decrease plasma hydrocortisone levels.

Methylprednisolone

Carbamazepine: Carbamazepine enhances the metabolism of methylprednisolone and can decrease plasma methylprednisolone levels.

Phenobarbital: Phenobarbital enhances the metabolism of methylprednisolone and can decrease plasma methylprednisolone levels.

Phenytoin: Phenytoin enhances the metabolism of methylprednisolone and can decrease plasma methylprednisolone levels.

Prednisolone

Carbamazepine: Carbamazepine enhances the metabolism of prednisolone and can decrease prednisolone elimination half-life values by ~ 28% and can increase prednisolone clearance by ~ 40%.

Phenobarbital: Phenobarbital enhances the metabolism of prednisolone and can increase prednisolone clearance by ~ 45%.

Phenytoin: Phenytoin enhances the metabolism of prednisolone and can decrease prednisolone elimination half-life values by 45% and can increase prednisolone clearance by 77%.

Oral contraceptives

Carbamazepine: Carbamazepine enhances the metabolism of oral contraceptives, thereby reducing the efficacy of the contraceptive pill and causing contraceptive failure. This loss of effectiveness relates to enhancement of the metabolism of the ethinyl estradiol and levonorgestrel components of oral contraceptives. Typically, ethinyl estradiol AUC values can decrease by ~42% and levonorgestrel AUC values can decrease ~ 58%.

Clonazepam: Clonazepam does not affect the metabolism of oral contraceptives.

Ethosuximide: Ethosuximide does not affect the metabolism of oral contraceptives.

Felbamate: Felbamate enhances the metabolism of oral contraceptives, thereby reducing the efficacy of the contraceptive pill and causing contraceptive failure. Typically, gestodene (progestin) AUC values can decrease by 42% and ethinyl estradiol AUC values can decrease by 13% after 30 days of felbamate therapy (1200mg twice daily).

Gabapentin: Gabapentin does not affect the metabolism of oral contraceptives.

Lamotrigine: Lamotrigine does not affect the metabolism of oral contraceptives.

Levetiracetam: Levetiracetam does not affect the metabolism of oral contraceptives.

Drug Interactions Between AEDs and Non-AED Drugs:

Oxcarbazepine: Oxcarbazepine enhances the metabolism of oral contraceptives, thereby reducing the efficacy of the contraceptive pill and causing contraceptive failure. This loss of effectiveness relates to induction of the metabolism of the ethinyl estradiol and levonorgestrel components of oral contraceptives. Typically, ethinylestradiol AUC values can decrease by 47% and levonorgestrel AUC values can decrease by 36%.

Phenobarbital: Phenobarbital enhances the metabolism of oral contraceptives, thereby reducing the efficacy of the contraceptive pill and causing contraceptive failure. This loss of effectiveness relates to induction of the CYP3A4-mediated metabolism of ethinylestradiol and levonorgestrel. Typically, ethinylestradiol and levonorgestrel AUC values can decrease by 40%.

Phenytoin: Phenytoin enhances the metabolism of oral contraceptives, thereby reducing the efficacy of the contraceptive pill and causing contraceptive failure. This loss of effectiveness relates to induction of the CYP3A4-mediated metabolism of ethinylestradiol and levonorgestrel. Typically, ethinylestradiol and levonorgestrel AUC values decrease by 50%.

Pregabalin: Pregabalin does not affect the metabolism of oral contraceptives.

Primidone: Primidone enhances the metabolism of oral contraceptives, thereby reducing the efficacy of the contraceptive pill and causing contraceptive failure. This loss of effectiveness relates to induction of the CYP3A4-mediated metabolism of ethinyl estradiol and levonorgestrel. Typically, ethinyl estradiol and levonorgestrel AUC values decrease by 40%.

Tiagabine: Tiagabine does not affect the metabolism of oral contraceptives.

Topiramate: Topiramate caused a 30% decline in plasma ethinyl estradiol levels but no change in norethindrone plasma levels in 12 women receiving a low-dose combination oral contraceptive. The mechanism for the reduction in plasma ethinyl estradiol levels is not known. The interaction is minimal or absent at topiramate daily dosages of 200 mg or less. Nevertheless, because contraceptive effectiveness may be affected, caution is advised in patients receiving topiramate and oral contraceptives.

STEROIDS

Valproic acid:	Valproic acid does not affect the metabolism of oral contraceptives.
Vigabatrin:	Vigabatrin does not affect the metabolism of oral contraceptives.
Zonisamide:	Zonisamide does not affect the metabolism of oral contraceptives.

Interactions Affected by AEDs

MISCELLANEA

Bupropion

Carbamazepine: Carbamazepine enhances the metabolism of bupropion and can decrease plasma bupropion levels. The implications of the interaction are unclear due to a concurrent increase in the plasma level of an active metabolite.

Phenobarbital: Phenobarbital enhances the metabolism of bupropion and can decrease plasma bupropion levels. The implications of the interaction are unclear due to a concurrent increase in the plasma level of an active metabolite.

Phenytoin: Phenytoin enhances the metabolism of bupropion and can decrease plasma bupropion levels. The implications of the interaction are unclear due to a concurrent increase in the plasma level of an active metabolite.

Primidone: Primidone enhances the metabolism of bupropion and can decrease plasma bupropion levels. The implications of the interaction are unclear due to a concurrent increase in the plasma level of an active metabolite.

Dihydroergotamine

Topiramate: Topiramate does not affect the pharmacokinetics of dihydroergotamine.

Local anaesthetics

Lidocaine (Lignocaine)

Carbamazepine: Carbamazepine enhances the metabolism of lidocaine, probably via an action on CYP3A4, and can decrease lidocaine AUC values by 60% and can increase lidocaine clearance 3-fold.

Phenobarbital: Phenobarbital enhances the metabolism of lidocaine, probably via an action on CYP3A4, and can decrease lidocaine AUC values by 60% and can increase lidocaine clearance 3-fold.

Phenytoin: Phenytoin enhances the metabolism of lidocaine, probably via an action on CYP3A4, and can decreases lidocaine AUC values by 60% and can increase lidocaine clearance 3-fold.

Primidone:	Primidone enhances the metabolism of lidocaine, probably via an action on CYP3A4, and can decrease lidocaine AUC values by 60% and can increase lidocaine clearance 3-fold.

Non-steroidal anti-inflammatory drugs
Diflunisal

Valproic acid:	Valproic acid does not affect the pharmacokinetics of diflunisal.

Naproxen

Valproic acid:	Valproic acid inhibits the metabolism of naproxen, via an action on glucuronidation and CYP2C9, and can decrease naproxen clearance by 10%.

Sumatriptan

Topiramate:	Topiramate enhances the clearance of sumatriptan by 9% and can decrease plasma sumatriptan levels by 11%.

Theophylline

Carbamazepine:	Carbamazepine enhances the metabolism of theophylline and can decrease theophylline elimination half-life values by 48%.
Phenobarbital:	Phenobarbital enhances the metabolism of theophylline and can increase theophylline clearance by up to 54%.
Phenytoin:	Phenytoin enhances the metabolism of theophylline and can increase theophylline clearance by up to 75%.

Anderson GD. A mechanistic approach to antiepileptic drug interactions. *Annals of Pharmacotherapy 1998; 32: 554-563.*

Andersson T. Pharmacokinetics, metabolism and interactions of acid pump inhibitors. Focus on omeprazole, lansoprazole and pantoprazole. *Clinical Pharmacokinetics 1996; 31: 9-28.*

Bertz RJ, Granneman GR. Use of in vitro and in vivo data to estimate the likelihood of metabolic pharmacokinetic interactions. *Clinical Pharmacokinetics 1997; 32: 210-258.*

Bialer M, Doose DR, Murthy B, Curtin C, Wang SS, Twyman RE, Schwabe S. Pharmacokinetic interactions of topiramate. *Clinical Pharmacokinetics 2004; 43: 763-780.*

Classen D, Pestonik, S, Evans S, Lloyd JF, Burke JP. Averse drug events in hospitalised patients. Excess length of stay, extra costs, and attributable mortality. *Journal of the American Medical Association 1997; 227: 301-306.*

Crawford P. Interactions between antiepileptic drugs and hormonal contraception. *CNS Drugs 2002; 16: 263-272.*

Fugh-Berman A. Herb-drug interactions. *Lancet 2000, 355: 134-138.*

Fuhr U. Induction of drug metabolizing enzymes: pharmacokinetic and toxicological consequences in humans. *Clinical Pharmacokinetics 2000; 38: 493-504.*

Hachad H, Ragueneau-Majlessi I, Levy RH. New antiepileptic drugs: review on drug interactions. *Therapeutic Drug Monitoring 2002; 24: 91-103.*

Ito K, Brown HS, Houston B. Database analyses for the prediction of in vivo drug-drug interactions from in vitro data. *British Journal of Clinical Pharmacology 2004; 57: 473-486.*

Johannesen SI. Plasma drug concentration monitoring of anticonvulsants. Practical guidelines. *CNS Drugs 1997; 7: 349-365.*

Johannesen SI, Battino D, Berry DJ, Bialer M, Kramer G, Tomson T, Patsalos PN. Therapeutic drug monitoring of the newer antiepileptic drugs. *Therapeutic Drug Monitoring 2003; 25: 347-363.*

Levy RH, Mattson RH, Meldrum BS, Perucca E, eds. *Antiepileptic Drugs,* 5th ed. New York, NY: Lippincott Williams & Wilkins, 2002.

Malaty LI, Kuper JJ. Drug interactions of HIV protease inhibitors. *Drug Safety 1999; 20: 147-169.*

May TW, Korn-Merker E, Rambeck B. Clinical pharmacokinetics of oxcarbazepine. *Clinical Pharmacokinetics 2003; 42: 1023-1042.*

Natsch S, Hekster YA, Keyser A, Deckers CLP, Meinardi H, Renier WO. Newer antiepileptic drugs: Role of pharmacology, drug interactions and adverse reactions in drug choice. *Drug Safety 1997; 17: 228-240.*

Nebert DW, Russell DW. Clinical importance of the cytochrome P450. *Lancet 2002; 360: 1155-1162.*

Patsalos PN. Levetiracetam: pharmacology and therapeutics in the treatment of epilepsy and other neurological conditions. *Reviews in Contemporary Pharmacotherapy 2004; 13: 1-168.*

Patsalos PN, Froscher W, Pisani F, van Rijn C. The importance of drug interactions in epilepsy therapy. *Epilepsia 2002; 43: 365-385.*

Patsalos PN, Perucca E. Clinically important drug interactions in epilepsy: general features and interactions between antiepileptic drugs. *Lancet Neurology 2003; 2: 347-356.*

Patsalos PN, Perucca E. Clinically important drug interactions in epilepsy: Interactions between antiepileptic drugs and other drugs. *Lancet Neurology 2003; 2: 473-481.*

Riva R, Albani F, Contin M, Baruzzi A. Pharmacokinetic interactions between antiepileptic drugs: Clinical considerations. *Clinical Pharmacokinetics 1996; 31: 470-493.*

Smith C. Drug interactions between psychoactive agents and antiepileptic agents. *Epilepsy & Behavior 2001; 2: 92-105.*

Spina E, Perucca E. Clinical significance of pharmacokinetic interactions between antiepileptic and psychoactive drugs. *Epilepsia 2002; 43 (Suppl. 2): 37-44.*

Spina E, Pisani F, Perucca E. Clinically significant pharmacokinetic interactions with carbamazepine: An update. *Clinical Pharmacokinetics 1996; 31: 198-214.*

Tanaka E. Clinically important pharmacokinetic drug-drug interactions: role of cytochrome P450 enzymes. *Journal of Clinical Pharmacy and Therapeutics 1998; 23: 403-416.*

Taburet AM, Singlas E. Drug interactions with antiviral drugs. *Clinical Pharmacokinetics 1996; 30: 385-401.*

Theis JGW, Koren G, Daneman R, Sherwin AL, Menzano E, Cortez M, Hwang P. Interactions of clobazam with conventional antiepileptics in children. *Journal of Child Neurology 1997; 12: 208-213.*

Tribut O, Lessard Y, Reymann J-M, Allain H, Bentue-Ferrer D. Pharmacogenomics. *Medical Science Monitor 2002; 8: RA152-RA163.*

Tyagi A, Delanty N. Herbal remedies, dietary supplements, and seizures. *Epilepsia 2003; 44: 228-235.*

Vecht CJ, Wagner GL, Wilms EB. Interactions between antiepileptic and chemotherapeutic drugs. *Lancet Neurology 2003; 2: 404-409.*

NOTES

NOTES

NOTES

NOTES

NOTES

NOTES

NOTES